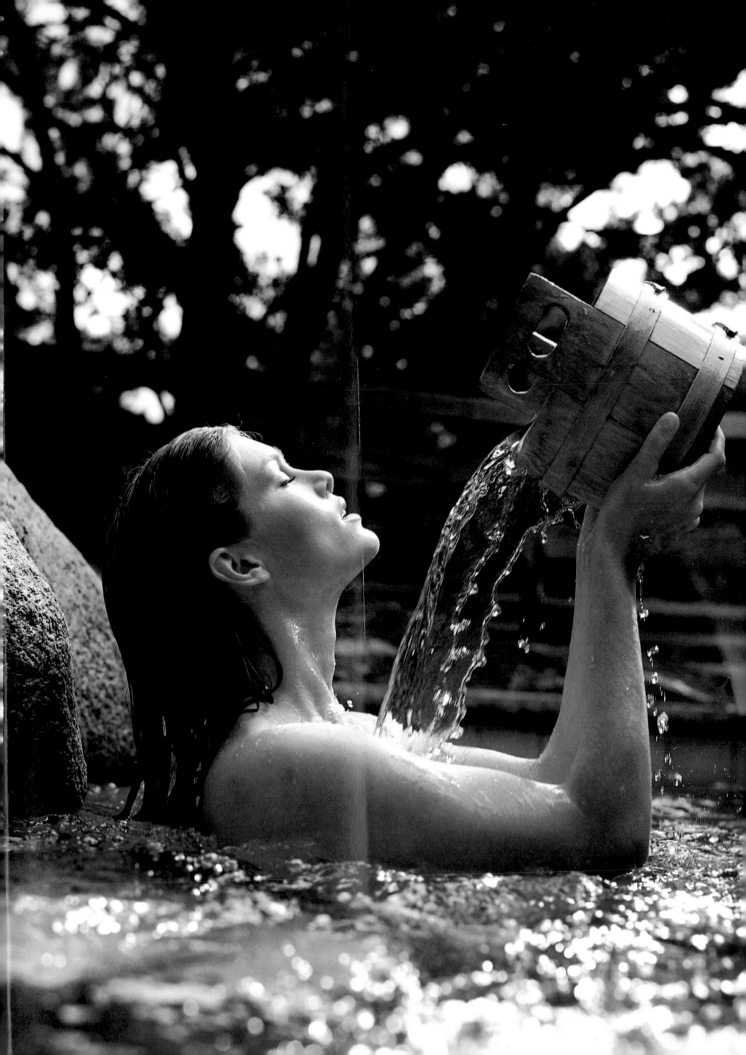

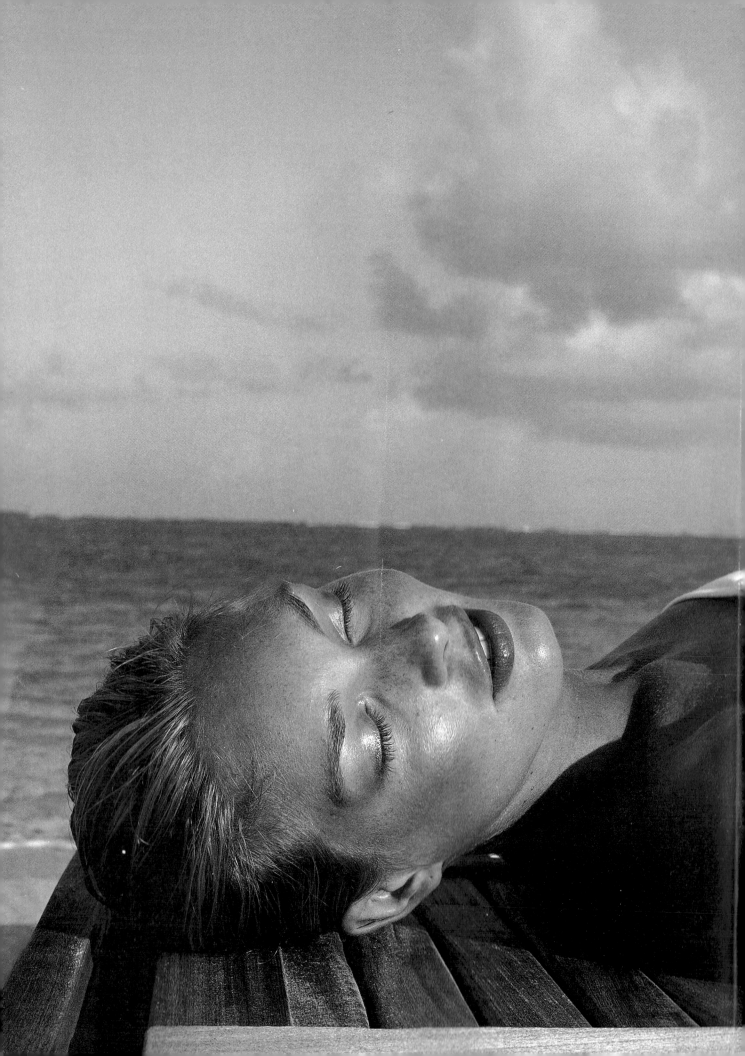

spa

PAMPER body and soul WITH

IDEAS FROM THE WORLD'S BEST SOURCES

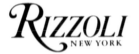

KARENA CALLEN

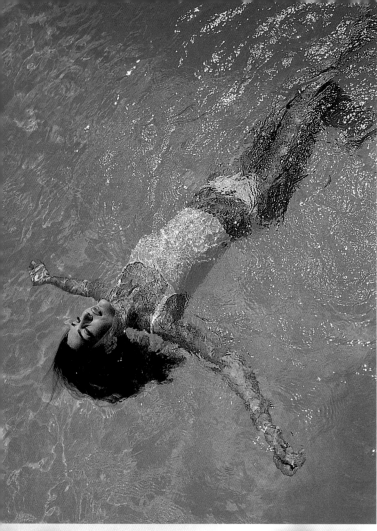

To my beautiful daughters, Shannon Emerald Georgia and Scarlet Alice Erin. Thank you for your love and for making me laugh.

First published in the United States of America in 2001 by
Rizzoli International Publications, Inc.
300 Park Avenue South
New York, NY 10010

Text © Karena Callen 2001

First published in the United Kingdom in 2001 by Ebury Press
Random House, 20 Vauxhall Bridge Road, London SW1V 2SA

ISBN 0-8478-2321-0
Library of Congress Catalog Card Number 00-111071

Editor: Emma Callery
Designer: Helen Lewis

Printed and bound in Singapore by Tien Wah Press

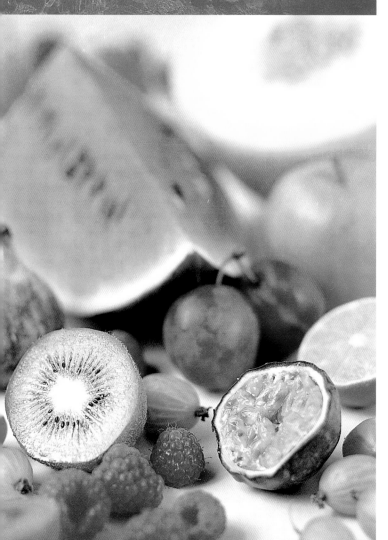

CONTENTS

So near, so spa

Spa: a tiny word that has grown in significance. No longer merely associated with mineral springs and therapeutic taking-of-the-waters, Roman baths, and Jane Austen, spa has taken on a new mantle that is hipper-than-hip. Be it in the form of to-die-for pampering products that line the shelves of the plushest beauty boutiques and most desirable department stores, mouth-watering and health-boosting cuisine, or the ultimate in holiday destinations, you can't get away from the "s" word these days.

For me, and a growing number of spa-goers, spa is the ultimate chill-out mantra. Personally, I only have to think it, to repeat it silently a few times in my head, and my blood pressure drops, my heart rate halves, and my muscles begin to soften and relax. It transports me back to my favorite spa resorts that I have been fortunate enough to visit during my fifteen years as a pampered and privileged health and beauty director on glossy magazines.

And for millions of devotees, spa means time out from the hardships of life, the hubbub of urban living, and the rigors of responsibility. Not only that, it is synonymous with peace, calm, tranquility, me-time, space, and getting-away-from-it-all. In fact, some fervent spa-worshippers are so devotional, that they have even gone as far as to suggest that "spas are the new churches."

HAVE IT YOUR OWN WAY

But while escapism is an all-important part of the spa concept, in reality, few of us have the time or bank balance to allow us to pack up and check in every time we reach crisis point. Spa resorts may offer a once-in-a-while retreat from the madness, but ultimately, creating a sanctuary within our own space is the key to long-term stress survival. As a mother of three and with a decreasing amount of time to spend on myself, I no longer have the time or money to languor in the lap of luxury in faraway spa resorts. The closest I get these days to pampering is a candlelit soak in the tub at the end of a long day. So I feel that I can speak from experience, as I've learned to make the most of a home-spa experience. And while my bathroom of the moment is a million miles away from my dream sanctuary, it's amazing what a soothing bath oil, a few scented tea lights, and a pile of fluffy towels can do.

Indeed, it's perfectly possible to recreate the ambience that you might find at reknowned spas such as Canyon Ranch or Chiva-Som in your own bathroom by bringing in essential spa elements–aromas, accessories, indulgent pampering recipes for face and body, cozy, plump towels, and sumptuous dressing gowns. They don't have to cost an arm and a leg.

It's this down-to-earth, practical philosophy that inspired this book. The tips, hints, recipes, and inspiration gathered from deluxe and dreamy spas around the world allow you to sample the food, treatments, and programs that are offered–and all within the comfort zone of your own home. Or, if you've picked this up following a spa stay, it's the perfect take-home treat that will inspire you to keep up the good work long after you've left the spa behind.

Karena Callen

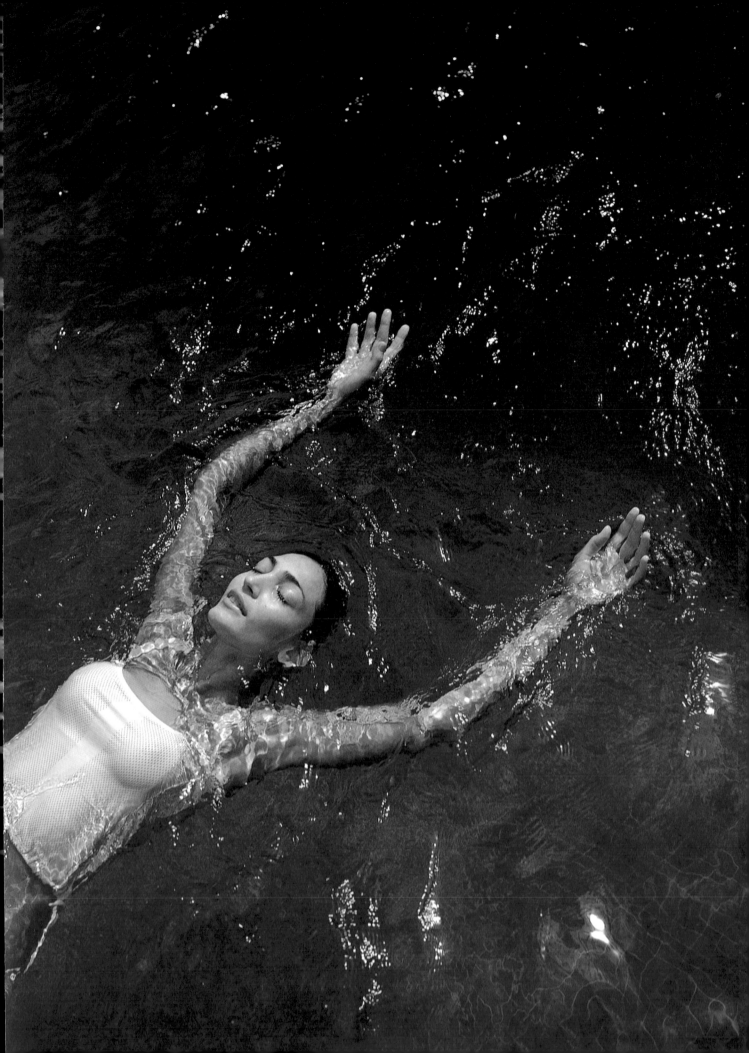

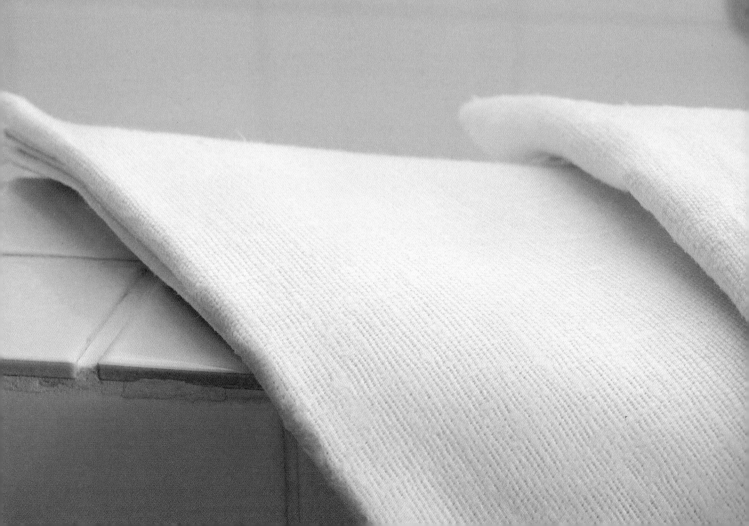

CREATING YOUR OWN
sanctuary

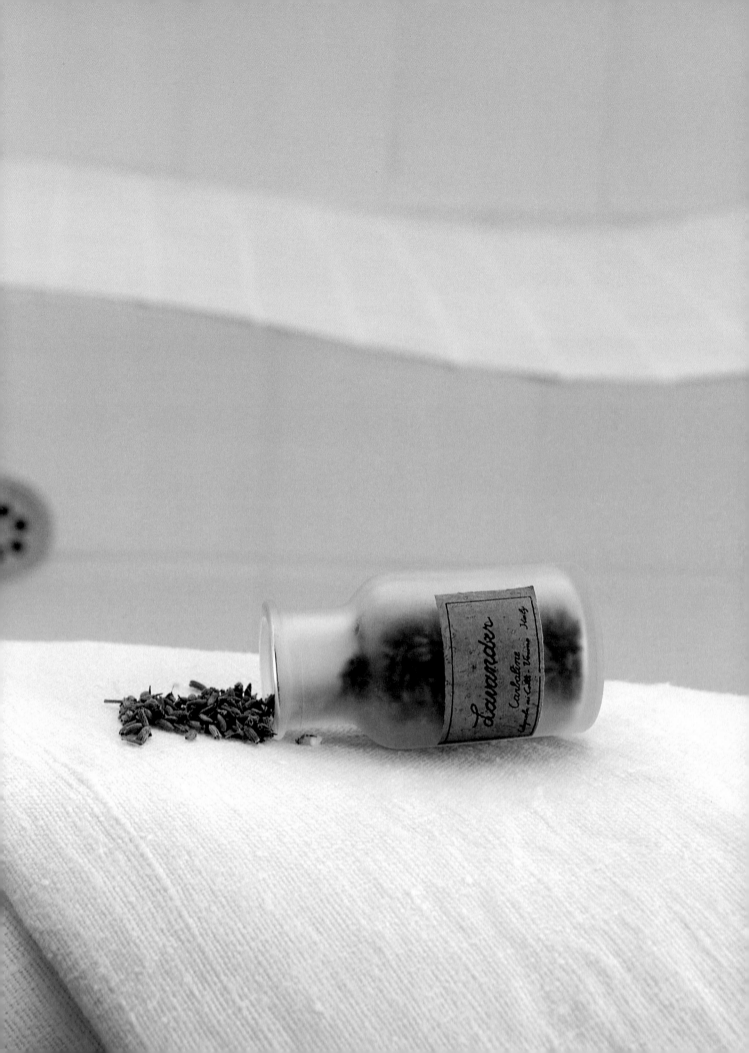

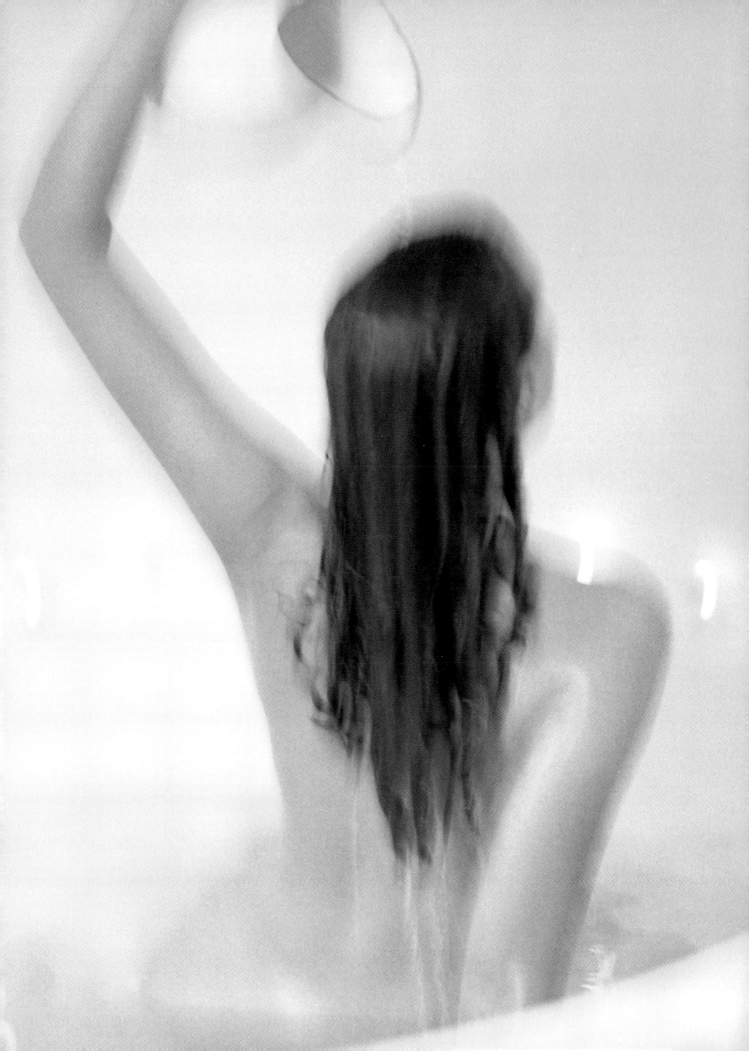

Comfort zone

We all need to retreat into our own private world from time to time, and–not surprisingly–most of us cite our bathroom as the ultimate chill-out zone. Of course, there's a good reason for this. Water and bathing have long been associated with relaxation and well being. From our own primeval connection to water to the fact that we all start out in a watery environment in the womb, you only have to look back at ancient cultures like the Egyptians, Greeks, and Romans to see the importance of cleansing mind, body, and spirit, and communing with water. For many of us, the sensation of being in water, of bathing and showering, is a sensual one. And as a result, the bathroom, where water flows in abundance, tends to be one of our favorite comfort zones. It's the closest environment to a spa that we have access to at home, the place where we can cocoon ourselves, hide away from the outside world, and get in touch with our most basic and natural needs. Not only that, but it is a realm where the majority of our senses can be pleasured. Textures, sounds, and aromas are plentiful in a well-stocked, well-planned bathroom.

While going to a spa ensures the right environment for detoxifying and unwinding, for most of us, it's a "once in a blue moon" treat. Our own bathroom, however, is always close at hand. The good news is that you can create a taste of what you will find at a spa at home–and the best news is that it doesn't mean you have to call in the architects and a posse of builders and plumbers either. "Small touches make all the difference," says Lydia Sarfati, founder of the beauty company Repechage. A pile of soft fluffy towels, a great wooden-handled body brush, or some aromatic candles can turn your plain old bathroom from dull to delicious in no time.

MINIMALIST DESIGN

Take a close look at the design of most spas and, no matter where they are in the world, one of the things you will notice is that they all tend to be uncluttered, pared-down, and minimalist. Ornaments are carefully chosen and the number limited to keep distractions to a minimum. This Zen-like approach can be seen at spas as far removed geographically as the Golden Door in California and Chiva-Som in Thailand. Comfort comes from essentials like soothing aromatic oils in sleek, glass bottles and over-sized cuddly robes that swaddle naked skin.

In addition to vital prerequisites like towels, slippers, and bathrobes, Sean Harrington, managing director of the beauty company Elemis and creator of over three hundred spas worldwide, cites lighting, music, stones, and pebbles as favorite home spa elements. "The perfect spa is a combination of elements that appeals to all the senses–music, lighting, textures, aromas–they all add up to create a harmonious environment." Think about having dimmer switches fitted so that you can lower the lights for additional intimacy, and stock up on candles. Lanterns and glass storm lights create soft, flickering light that will help to put you into a state of deep relaxation. Aromas are also essential in creating your home spa retreat. Choose the aromas to suit your mood, whether you want to be calm, perk yourself up, or encourage deep sleep.

Calming color

The colors that you use in creating your sanctuary can go a long way to improving your mood and, according to color therapists, can even help to stimulate your immune system and protect against illness. Using color to lift the spirits is hardly a new idea but one that more and more of us are absorbing into our everyday lives. Color therapy is no longer the staple of alternative health practitioners—it has been readily adopted by everyone from beauty companies to interior designers.

WHITES

From the chalkiest of whites to creamier calico and canvas tones, white creates a feeling of space, light, and purity, perfect for a spa-like environment. It will brighten dark spaces and spruce up and freshen a worn-out interior. White is a theme adopted at some of the most heavenly spa retreats. The Philippe Stark-designed spas, Agua at Delano in Miami and more recently at Agua at Sanderson in London, have been created using celestial shades of white from the crispest brilliant white to the softest wax white. The result is a feeling of spaciousness, described by co-creator Leila Fazel as "if you're floating on a cloud." Paint walls, ceilings, and woodwork with matte or eggshell paint in different hues of white. Give plain, sanded floorboards a new lease on life with white paint. Dress windows with billowing white muslin or white shutters.

BLUES

Being the color of water and sky, blue always has a feel-good association. Used in many spas to create a sense of calm and relaxation, on a practical level, light translucent blues can also help to attract light into a dark room. From the palest of baby blues to more vibrant hyacinth or bluebell, blue brings with it a seaside, holiday feel and works well in the context of a bathroom. Deeper Moroccan-style cobalt and lapis blues can be teamed with mosaic wall tiles and terracotta floor tiles to create an exotic oasis.

GREENS

For a spa-style space, choose the palest, most light reflective greens and team them with fresh white, terracotta, or sun-drenched yellow. On a spiritual note, green is the color of the heart chakra. It is a famously soothing, harmonious color that creates a natural environment. For a stronger statement, go for bolder shades such as turquoise and lime. Greens work well with natural wood or bamboo bathroom accessories and plain white baths and sinks. Recreate the tranquility at Chiva-Som International Health Resort, Thailand, by using a combination of turquoise mosaic tiles, dark wooden accessories, pale green walls, and potted palms and grasses.

VIOLET AND LAVENDER

Violet and lavender are often chosen because of their light attracting and purifying properties. In spiritual terms, violet is the color of the "third eye"—located in the center of our brow—and is a truly sedative color that helps to calm the central nervous system. Violet also helps us to tune in to our more intuitive side and therefore enables us to successfully access our higher consciousness.

Choose from the palest wash of lilac to stronger violets for a soothing, modern sanctuary. This spectrum of colors looks best with clean, simple accessories such as chrome, stainless steel, and pale blonde wood. Classic, timeless objects such as a fifties Arne Jacobsen butterfly chair look perfect against lilacs and lavenders.

YELLOWS

Like white, yellow helps open up dingy, dark rooms and creates the illusion of space and light. Uplifting and awakening, sunny yellows always work as a mood enhancer and bring a sense of clarity and mental focus when used in room decoration. Incidentally, yellow relates to the solar plexus chakra, located just below the sternum.

Choose from creamy, buttery tones, vibrant egg yolk shades, and deep mustards. Yellows and creams complement each other perfectly, creating a sunny, rustic feel. To complete the look, add simple pine or painted wood accessories, piles of soft, fluffy towels, and canvas roman blinds or painted wooden shutters.

ORANGES

From the palest peach through to brilliant tangerine, the orange palette will warm up a cold space and make it feel cozier. Orange is the color that represents the sacral chakra—just below the navel—the center of pleasure and well being, so it's a very positive shade with which to surround yourself.

For a sensual sanctuary, combine it with terracotta tiles, simple earthenware containers, and slatted wooden blinds for a feel that's similar to the Vista Clara Ranch Resort and Spa in New Mexico. Or conjure up an environment reminiscent of the Nusa Dua Spa in Bali by teaming orange with egg yolk yellow or dark green, and adding dark wood or bamboo fixtures and fittings, as well as simple glass bottles and jars filled with bath and body oils. Complete the mood by burning sandalwood or jasmine incense.

REDS

Red is not a relaxing color, although darker shades can make a room feel cozy. Red represents the root chakra, located in the pelvic region, and is associated with passion, sexual energy, and strength. If you do choose reds for your sanctuary stick to terracotta reds and deeper tones, and steer clear of vivid or tomato reds. Shades of terracotta predominate at Rancho La Puerta in Mexico. Teamed with other vibrant shades like strong, deep pink, egg yolk yellow, and cobalt blue and natural materials like stripped wood, you can create a Rancho feel in your own sanctuary. Look out for Mexican-style pottery and tiles to complete the look.

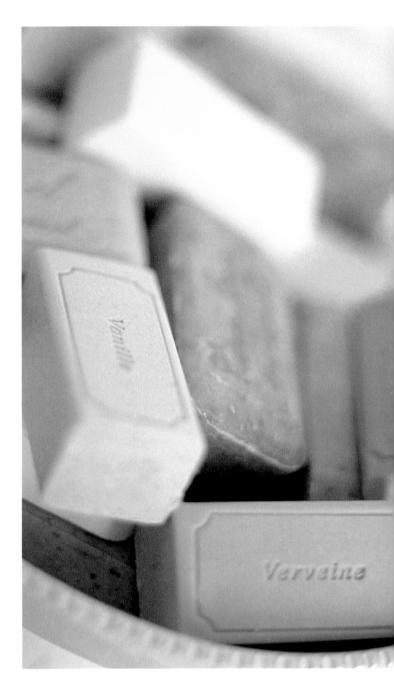

Aromas

Scent has the power to transport us not only to other times in our lives but to faraway places–destinations that we may have visited in reality or merely in our dreams. Each spa that I have visited has its own distinctive aroma that when smelled even years after, takes me back to my time spent there. In particular, Ten Thousand Waves in Santa Fe, New Mexico, emits the most wonderful mix of cedar and sage, native to that part of the state–one sniff of either and I am floating in a hot tub under the stars. Burning oils or incense in your bathroom will help you to create your own little temple, a space that is sacred to you and your family. This might be just the opportunity you need to remind yourself of a favorite spa or vacation, in which case, choose a scent that conjures images of that place.

LAVENDER

Always reminiscent of Provence, lavender is a clean, fresh scent that has potent relaxing properties. Hang bunches of dried lavender in linen cupboards to scent your towels and laundry, or burn lavender essential oil or scented candles in your bathroom to create a wonderful summer breeze through the room.

YLANG YLANG

One of the most popular essential oils used in tropical spas such as the Nusa Dua Spa in Bali, ylang ylang is renowned for its anti-depressant properties. It is also a powerful aphrodisiac. Ylang ylang combines well with woody aromas such as vetiver and also with sensual essential oils like jasmine and rose.

JASMINE

Used in profusion in Southeast Asian spas, jasmine has incredibly uplifting and sensual properties. Add a few drops of jasmine oil to your bath, burn it in an oil burner or, if you can track one down, bathe by the light of a jasmine scented candle. Sheer bliss.

PATCHOULI

For some, patchouli brings back too many memories of the hippy trail, but for others it is one of the most arousing, sexy fragrances. Popular in many of the Malaysian and Balinese spas, it is used not only as a perfume and room scent but to treat skin conditions as diverse as eczema and acne. Use in small doses or you could find your loved ones leaving home. Patchouli incense creates the most wonderful earthy aroma conducive to a meditative state.

SAGE

One of my favorite aromas at home, sage is a real cleanser. Part of many Native American ceremonies, it is often used in the form of smudge sticks–tightly bound bundles of sage–that are set alight and then snuffed out. The smoke is used to rid a room of any bad vibes. If you like the smell of sage, grow some in terracotta pots and keep that in your bathroom. Otherwise, you can find sage-based room fragrances, oils, and incense.

SANDALWOOD

Inhaling sandalwood is like stepping into a souk in Marrakech or a Southeast Asian spa.

Sandalwood has been used for centuries in purification rituals and is said to have potent mind and body relaxing properties. Sandalwood oil is used at many of the Asian spas, particularly in massage, and is also very good for re-balancing oily skin (see the facial blends given on page 100). Burn the essential oil or buy it in incense form for a traditional sandalwood experience.

EUCALYPTUS

A favorite with Australian spas, eucalyptus has a wonderful medicinal aroma that really clears sinuses and helps to fight off colds and flu. Team this particular oil with tea tree oil for a really traditional Antipodean rescue remedy. Eucalyptus also works very well in the shower. Put a few drops on a sponge and then vigorously massage it into your skin as you shower.

TEA TREE

Another favorite with Australian spas, tea tree has powerful antiseptic properties and is a great room purifier. Mix tea tree with a little peppermint, eucalyptus, and lavender for a deep-cleansing effect. Add a few drops to a vaporizer or bowl of warm water.

CEDARWOOD

Popular at southwestern spas in the United States, cedarwood is excellent for boosting flagging energy levels and low self-esteem. It works well in combination with sandalwood, ylang ylang, sage, and jasmine. Put a few drops in an oil burner or on a damp cotton wool ball placed behind a radiator for a woody, outdoorsy aroma.

SCENTING YOUR SANCTUARY

Create different moods by hand-blending your own essential oil combinations.

Purification: If you are in need of a detox, try this blend of cleansing oils. Add 2 drops of tea tree oil to 3 drops of eucalyptus and 2 drops of peppermint. Put into an oil burner or vaporizer to purify your sanctuary. This blend is also perfect for chasing away colds and flu. Tea tree is an excellent antiseptic, while eucalyptus helps to clear the nasal passages, and peppermint can help to reduce a temperature.

Sacred space: When you need to retreat and cocoon yourself, blend 3 drops of lavender with 2 drops of sage and 2 drops of frankincense, and add to 1 tablespoon of a carrier oil such as aloe vera or avocado oil. Add to a warm bath just as you step into it. The aroma will fill the room too, leaving you feeling cozy and nurtured.

Chill out: Burning the candle at both ends? Living life in the fast lane and can't put on the brakes? Surround yourself with this blend to bring you back to a slower, steadier pace. Add 5 drops of lavender to 4 drops of patchouli, 3 drops of rose, and 3 drops of chamomile. Add to an oil burner to scent the room or to a bowl of steaming water and inhale for a few minutes. To make your own room scent, add a few drops of each oil to an atomizer containing distilled water and spray in the room, on to your bathrobe, and on to your pillow.

Laughter: When life is getting you down, use this uplifting blend to boost your spirits. Combine 4 drops of rose with 4 drops of tangerine, 2 drops of geranium, and 2 drops of bergamot and add to an oil burner or a small bowl of warm water placed on or near a radiator. The aroma will bring back your sense of humor.

Fixtures and fittings

One of the things the designs of the majority of spas have in common is that they are often pared-down and minimalist. Furthermore, there is that wonderful sense of freedom that comes from not being surrounded by all the clutter of home life. Comfort comes from elements like oils for massage, cozy toweling robes, and flickering candles. "Comfort is crucial," says international spa creator and managing director of beauty company E'Spa, Susan Harmsworth. "Investing in simple but luxurious accessories and storage containers to keep things ordered ensures that your space looks crisp and clean. You won't have to spend your valuable relaxation time having to move things around or rummaging for that favorite body cream."

SIMPLE STORAGE

There is a huge difference between a spa and a home, but in terms of achieving a spa look, clearing away clutter is key. Keep an eye out for elegant glass jars in which to keep essential prerequisites like cotton balls and cotton swabs. Stainless steel or metallic canisters look orderly and give a modern feel to a plain wooden shelf or window sill, while hand-made Shaker wooden boxes offer a more rustic option, especially when teamed with generous wicker laundry baskets.

When it comes to cupboards, search antique shops and flea markets for old-style cabinets that can be painted with eggshell paint to match walls and woodwork. Hotel-style chrome trolleys are both stylish and ergonomic, as they can be easily moved around when stocked with favorite bathing essentials and piles of soft, fluffy towels and flannels.

TOWEL RAILS

Whether you choose sleek chrome hotel-style towel rails or simple New Mexican inspired wooden towel ladders, a place to hang your towels close to the bath is a real essential. Heated towel rails are particularly worth investing in, especially for winter, when there really is nothing so appealing as wrapping your body in a plush, warm towel.

Alternatively, you can prop a simple wooden rail against the wall over an existing radiator to ensure that your towels and bathrobe are warmed up. Or consider painting wooden towel rails to do a similar job.

BEAUTIFUL BATHS

From luxurious, break-the-bank Japanese-style wooden tubs hewn out of aromatic cedar to cast iron junkyard finds, the perfect bath depends entirely on your own taste. Given the choice, I'd go for a free-standing, Victorian-style cast iron tub any day. I love the vast, deep space and the fact that I can have a pile of books at one side and a table with scented candles and a battery-operated CD player and radio for essential soothing music on the other.

Whichever bath you choose, make sure you invest in a decent plumbing and water heating system to ensure that you have a constant, copious supply of hot water. There's nothing worse than having to wait for your bath to run or finding that you have three drops of hot water when you are craving a luxurious soak. The initial expense may be greater, but if it makes for longer-term relaxation it is worth it.

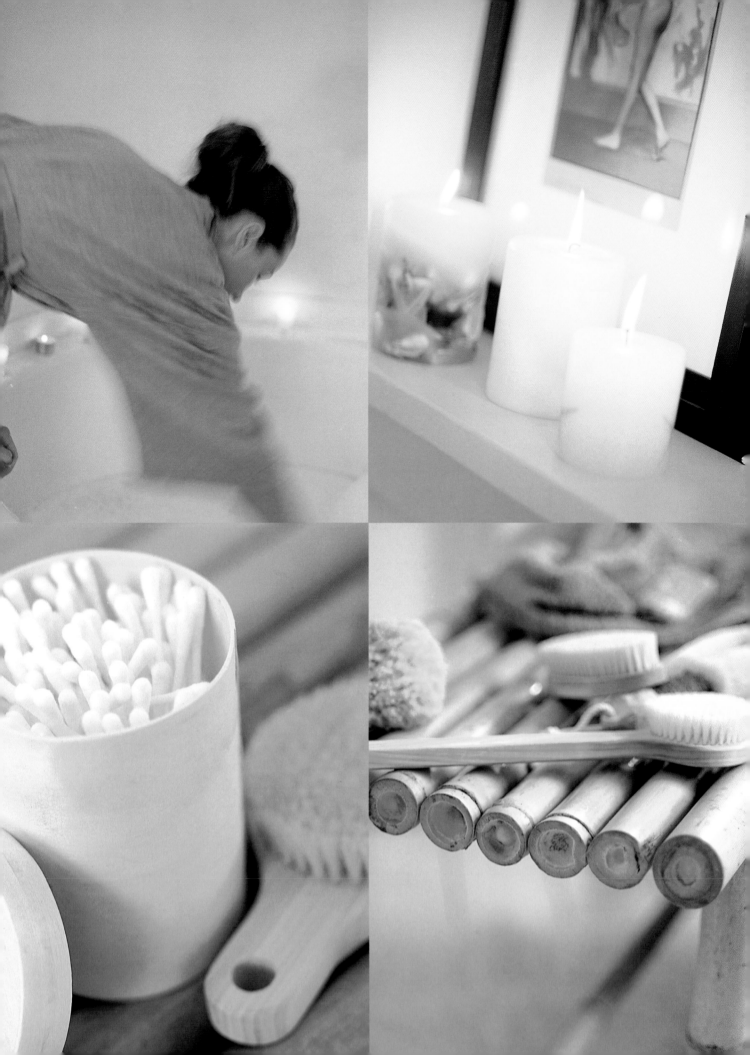

POWER SHOWERS

There's nothing more invigorating than starting the day under a stream of gorgeous, skin cleansing water, delivered at high pressure from an efficient shower. If you live in an area where the water pressure is low, a power shower is by far the best option, unless you want to find yourself standing under a feeble trickle of water that alternates hot and cold. If you enjoy a real soak, look for a shower with a large, chrome head, almost like an enormous watering can, which delivers a wonderful waterfall-like cascade. For those who prefer high-pressure needle-like jets, compact American-style six-prong showerheads are the best option.

MATERIAL CHOICES

• Toughened glass sinks with chrome fittings will enhance any modern, minimalist sanctuary.
• Stainless steel is both functional and streamline, although it may need to be treated with extra care to avoid scratching. It can look a little clinical, but works well with white woodwork and softer touches like blonde wooden accessories.
• Ceramic sinks can be found in a variety of shapes and sizes from square Belfast-style basins to modern, sculpted sinks. Easy to keep clean, they always look pure and pristine.
• Natural and reconstructed marble basins work well with dark, Japanese-style woods, such as mahogany and teak, and simple, streamlined accessories. Reconstructed marble basins are made by combining powdered marble and resin, and tend to be more durable than natural marble.

SPA AND WHIRLPOOL BATHS

If you have the opportunity and the budget for a complete bathroom makeover, putting in a spa or whirlpool bath will make even more of the time spent in your private sanctuary. Choose from spa baths that pump warm air into the bath water, whirlpool baths that re-circulate the water, or whirlpool spas that circulate a combination of water and air.

Choose from large, hot-tub-style circular baths to more traditional roll-top shapes and ensure that you have space for the pump, which needs to be installed either directly under the bath or in a storage cupboard. Spa baths do need to be installed by an expert and you will need to check that all electrical components are protected by a circuit breaker.

BASINS AND SINKS

Whether you opt for a basic porcelain sink or a high tech stainless steel basin, ensure that you invest in one that suits your everyday needs. In addition to being decorative, your basin should be practical—deep enough to allow you to dunk your hands and face if you need to and to ensure that you don't end up with a waterlogged floor. Take your pick from pedestal, wall-hung, or countertop styles, depending on the look you're after. In terms of materials, again the world's your oyster (see material choices, left).

Taps are also important—they need to be functional, not just decorative. Again, it is a matter of choice what style you pick and the variety is truly awe inspiring. Choose from traditional pillar-style, basin mixer, or single lever monobloc taps. Putting new taps on an old sink can smarten it up instantly.

Step into the light

Lighting is crucial in helping to create the right atmosphere in your sanctuary. From downlighters to candles, task lighting to spotlights, choosing the kind of illumination you want depends entirely on personal taste and individual needs.

Brilliant, blazing light is not an essential in a bathroom sanctuary. In fact, many types of artificial lighting can be cold and unflattering, so make the most of natural light during the day by choosing a color scheme that is light reflective and ensuring that window coverings are as translucent as possible. I don't care what any design gurus say about the modernity of fluorescent lighting–it's incredibly cold and unforgiving. If you want to create a really intimate, soothing environment, fluorescent lighting is best avoided altogether.

NATURAL LIGHT
Having a bathroom with windows and natural light will make life a lot easier. You can manipulate the light coming in by your choice of window treatments. Shutters and Venetian blinds allow privacy while letting daylight filter through. Opaque glass or transparent, gauzy curtains again give an element of privacy while allowing light to come through.

AMBIENT LIGHT
Nothing creates a more soothing, relaxing atmosphere than candlelight. For the ultimate in relaxing bath-time pampering, candlelight is hard to beat. Invest in a dozen or so little tea lights or dinner lights in glass containers and place them around your bath or on shelves around the room,

ensuring they are not near anything that's flammable. Large pillar candles also throw a beautiful light that's perfect for bathing by.

OVERALL LIGHTING
By far the most pleasing form of overall lighting, halogen downlighters cast an even, pure light over a room and can be dimmed for a softer effect and combined with candlelight in the evening. In addition, because they can be recessed into the ceiling, they don't intrude decoratively. Perfect for creating a modern, minimalist haven.

TASK LIGHTING
Spotlights and mirror lights provide a clear, direct light source and are a necessity, particularly if you are performing grooming acts such as eyebrow tweezing or applying make-up. Have them put on a separate switch to your main bathroom lighting so that they can be turned on only when you need them.

TIPS
• While aesthetics are obviously key when picking bathroom lighting, safety is paramount. Ensure that the lights you choose are suitable for bathroom use before fitting them. And for extra security, use a qualified electrician.
• Ceiling lights should be sealed within a plastic steam or waterproof diffuser.
• Avoid fitting wall-mounted light switches within your bathroom and opt instead for pull-cord fittings. Better still, place light switches outside the room.

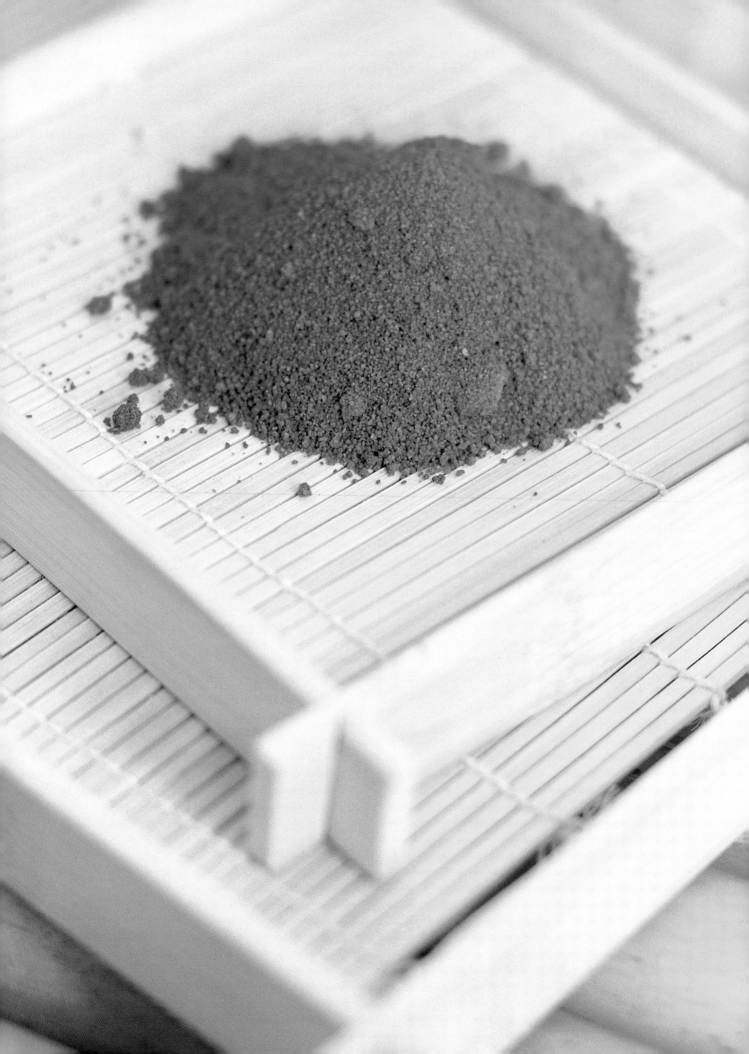

Textures

While the appearance and aroma of your sanctuary are crucial in creating a haven that's your own, never forget that the sense of touch is of the utmost importance. The feel of the objects that you choose for your bathroom can improve the quality of your time spent luxuriating. Textures can be complementary–the warmth of a wooden floor, piles of huge, fluffy bath sheets, rounded weathered glass storage jars and bottles –or you can choose to put opposites together for an equally pleasing sensation. Cool, smooth limestone flooring teamed with a soft, looped towelling bath mat or a weathered wooden duckboard work beautifully together. Billowy muslin curtains, teamed with plain white-washed plaster walls and piles of hand-picked pebbles from beach-combing trips please not only your eyes but your hands, as you explore the different textures while in your sanctuary.

ROUGH AND READY

Roughness is not a texture that immediately springs to mind in association with a sanctuary. But many natural materials are conducive to a peaceful, calming environment–think pumice, sisal, coir–and are often irregular and rough to the touch. The trick is to combine the rough with the smooth to create a rounded, textural experience that combines as many pleasurable sensations as possible. Roughly hewn stone jars and shallow bowls are perfect storage containers for bath salts, piles of scented, hand-made soaps, and collections of shells and driftwood. A sisal mat or runner feels stimulating under foot after a long soak in the tub. You can also transform a bland or featureless room by adding salvaged tongue-and-groove panelling or by choosing weather-beaten accessories such as a distressed painted wooden chair or cupboard.

SMOOTH

Rounded objects and smooth surfaces beg to be caressed and enjoyed. Especially suited to the bathroom, smooth textures–from polished limestone flooring to a marble fireplace, piles of sandblasted cobbles, and gently curved glass jars and bottles–are a pleasure to hold and touch. Spherical objects, like marbles and pebbles, look beautiful displayed in glass jars or in smooth, shallow bowls and can be used as meditation tools. Simply roll two large marbles or rounded pebbles between your fingers or in your palm as you relax in a warm bath. Close your eyes and focus on the rolling action to soothe away stress. Heap bars of smooth, aromatic soaps into bowls and jars to add color and texture.

Smooth floors, like limestone and marble, also feel and look clean in a bathroom–but be aware that they can be slippery when wet. Keep a wooden duckboard or absorbent bath mat at hand for post-bath safety.

SOFT

Nothing compares to the luxurious sensation of being swathed in a soft, thick-piled towel or robe after bathing. It takes us back to our childhood, makes us feel warm and secure and, on a practical note, dries us quickly. Stockpile jumbo-sized bath sheets, robes, and terry cloth bath slippers and store them in an airing cupboard for extra comfort. Replace your towels on a regular basis–old towels tend to become threadbare and lose their softness. Seek out the plushest, velour towels that are ideal for children, as they tend to have a more velvety texture than traditional looped towelling. Keep a plentiful supply of skin softening and soothing body oils, creams and lotions for post-bath massage–nothing feels more relaxing than a rub down.

Accessories

To make the most of your home spa, stock up on versatile accessories that not only look beautiful decoratively, but that enhance skin, mood, and your immediate environment. Fill a shallow wooden bowl with natural sponges or piles of multi-colored handmade soaps; hang body brushes on a simple Shaker-style peg rail, and stockpile fine muslin cloths and washcloths in a wire-fronted bathroom cupboard for easy access.

SPONGES
Skin has more affinity with natural sponges than with synthetic ones. Use them with soap or a favorite bath foam to achieve a sensual lather. A tip to prolong the life of a natural sponge is to soak it in vinegar once in a while. This will literally pickle and preserve it. Always make sure you rinse it well after bathing or showering and place it somewhere warm to dry.

BODY BRUSHES
Sisal and bristle body brushes can be hung up on hooks and peg rails, being both practical and ornamental. Body brushing is recommended by many therapists to stimulate the body's lymphatic system–basically a kind of waste disposal. When stressed, the lymphatic system can become sluggish, and a daily session of skin brushing–where you brush lightly across dry skin with a body brush, always working toward the heart–is thought to be beneficial.

LOOFAHS
Excellent for scrubbing parts that are tricky to reach, fibrous loofahs help to stimulate the circulation and exfoliate the skin, and generally work a bit like a natural steel wool pad. They need to be rinsed and dried to preserve them.

MUSLIN CLOTHS AND WASHCLOTHS
Best for cleansing sensitive skin, muslin cloths and washcloths exfoliate gently and when combined with a cleansing oil or cream, they are super effective skin polishers. If the skin on your face is acting up and misbehaving, soak a muslin cloth in very hot water to which a few drops of tea tree and lavender essential oils are added and then place over your face as you relax in a warm bath.

PUMICE STONES
With its neutral color and organic texture, pumice stone blends in equally well with a very modern or rustic-style sanctuary. Ideal for polishing away hard skin on feet, especially heels, pumice comes in a variety of shapes and sizes.

BATH AND SEA SALTS
Fill glass apothecary and flip-top preserve jars with all kinds of sea and bath salts. Not only are they perfect for creating instant skin-softening body scrubs when mixed with a little oil, they add color and texture to the bathroom environment.

PEBBLES AND COBBLES
Beach-combed pebbles and cobbles not only look beautiful piled on shelves and on the floor– they can be used for massage too. Warm them in hot water with a little oil, and use them to massage hands and feet while soaking in the bath.

CHILL-OUT MUSIC

Music is one of the most powerful mediums that you can use to transport you from the real world to your own personal Nirvana. Tune in to sounds that will help you release tension and bottled-up emotions.

Arabesque

A compilation by Momo (Gut Records)

Guaranteed to chase away the blues, this up-tempo, North African chill-out music will make you smile rather than sleep. Put this on after a hard day at the office and you'll find yourself transported to exotic locations without having to leave the coziness of your own sanctuary.

Astral Weeks

by Van Morrison (Warner Brothers)

Stunningly beautiful lyrics and melodies paint dreamy pictures that will leave you feeling completely "at one" with the universe.

Big Calm

by Morcheeba (Indochina Records)

Modern chill-out music at its best—and not a twangy sound or dolphin click in evidence. If you hate the grating New Age music passed off as relaxing, you'll love this. Soak in the tub and relax with a face mask.

Divine Bliss

by Shri Anandi Ma (Sounds True)

Blissful Indian devotional music that will help you to achieve your own trance-like state. Perfect for meditation.

Gone to Earth

by David Sylvian (Virgin Records)

Deeply soothing songs to take you to another world that's far from the stressful one you currently inhabit. One to listen to while you wallow in the bath.

The Moon and the Melodies

by Harold Budd, Simon Raymonde, Robin Guthrie, and Elizabeth Fraser (4AD)

Be prepared to be lulled and tranquilized by tantalizing vocals and wonderful, ethereal melodies. The perfect soothe-you-to-sleep sounds.

The Pearl

by Harold Budd and Brian Eno (EG Records)

Unlock pent-up tension by playing this deliciously composed ambient treasury. Better than any lullaby, put it on and you'll be soothed into a state of total tranquility.

Southern Exposure

by Alex de Grassi (Windham Hill Records)

Here is gorgeous solo guitar that takes you to sun-filled landscapes and big skies with billowing clouds. Perfect for curling up with on your beanbag and soaking up those sounds for a thorough wind-down.

Spirit Horses: The Music of James DeMars

by R. Carlos Nakai (Canyon)

Eerie and beautiful, this Native American flute music, as recommended by Westward Look Resort in Arizona, will carry you to another plain of consciousness. The ideal accompaniment to yoga or meditation.

Symphonies 40 and 38

by Mozart, performed by the English Chamber Orchestra (Decca)

Guaranteed to lift your mood and divert your attention from the hassles of everyday life.

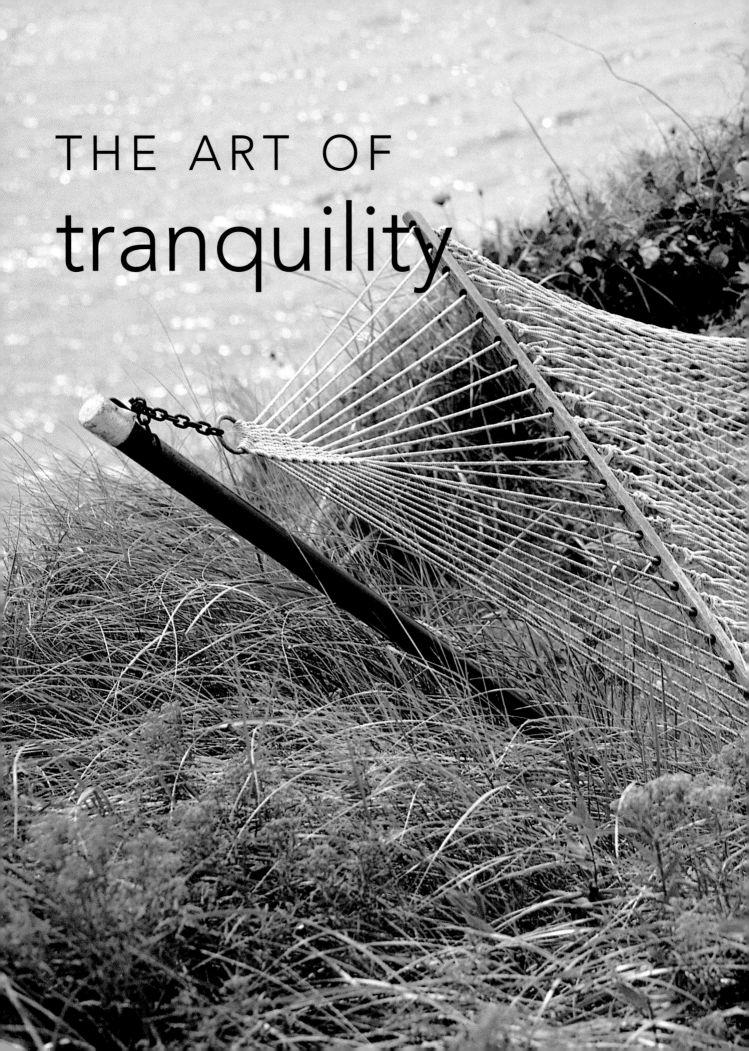

THE ART OF
tranquility

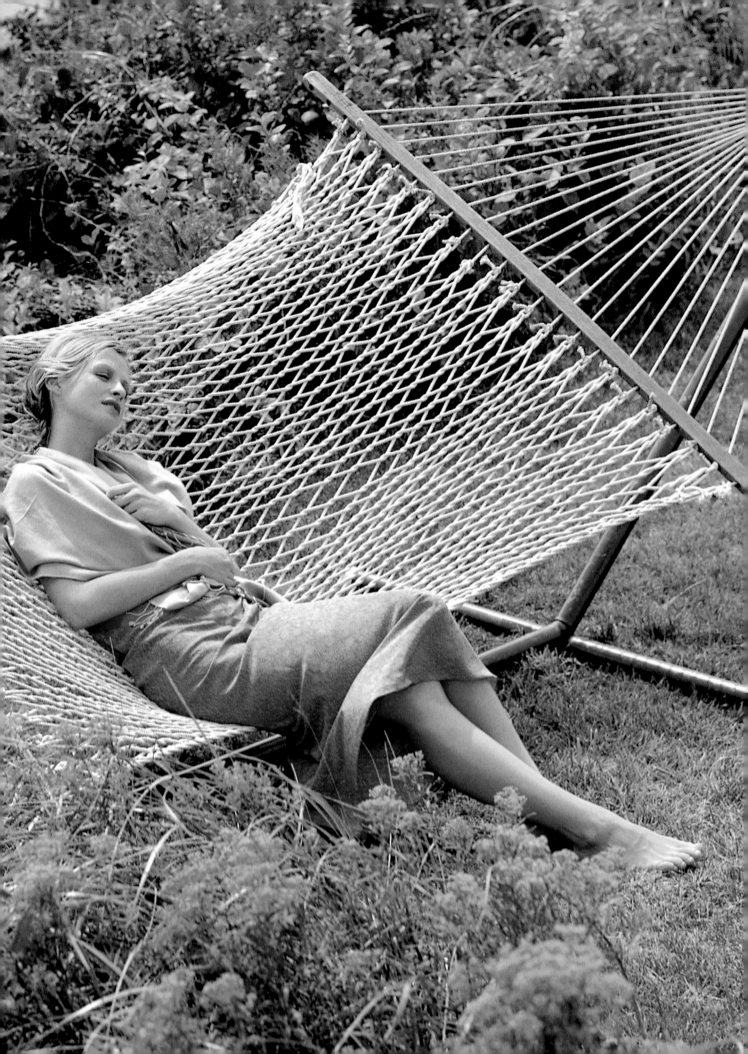

Learn to relax

If I ever do have the chance to book a spa vacation, my motivation could be summed up by the desperate need for one thing–relaxation. Peace, calm, tranquility–call it what you will, there is just not enough of this precious commodity in our modern, stress-filled lives. We are all guilty of doing too much, biting off more than we can chew, and running on empty. But all too often we are so busy running to stand still, that we do not stop to think of the consequences. Burn-out, fatigue, stress-related illnesses, and insomnia are all the result of overload.

THE STRESS FACTOR

Of course, we all need an element of stress in our lives in order to function, otherwise we would probably just curl up on the sofa and refuse to move. Deadlines, financial pressures, and the demands of family and friends all motivate us in both positive and negative ways. We all get wrapped up in our own stress cycles and become so accustomed to the physical and emotional demands that stress puts on us, that we become accustomed to living under stress. In physical terms, this eventually takes its toll. The reason? When we are under stress, be it stuck in a traffic jam or on a job interview, our bodies undergo physiological changes. Adrenaline races through our veins, raising our cortisol levels–one of the main stress hormones. As a result, our energy levels soar–in primitive times this fight or flight response fuelled our ability to defend ourselves from predators or, if we saw fit, to run away super fast. But just as energy levels rise and our heart beats rapidly, we fall into a vicious cycle of highs and lows. Eventually, our adrenal glands can become fatigued and thyroxin–a hormone that controls our metabolism–becomes depleted, leaving us feeling exhausted and without any *joie de vivre*. An all-too-familiar scenario for a growing number of us.

THE ANTI-STRESS SPA SOLUTION

Enough gloom. There is a simple solution to this modern dilemma, and that is to follow the pathway that the ancient cultures laid down in order to keep life in balance and to stay free of disease. That is, to learn the art of tranquility, to relax, to do nothing, to chill out or, to be calm, to contemplate–basically, to return our minds and bodies to a Zen-like state. This may be easier said than done, yet it is not as difficult or monumental as you might think. The secret is to take up a specific technique that allows you to unwind. Transcendental meditation is my own particular key whereas for others more active methods such as t'ai chi, yoga, or aikido will do the trick. It's all down to finding out what suits your physical and emotional needs and this is often a case of trial and error.

Relaxation techniques are a growing part of spa culture with practices like yoga and t'ai chi becoming more and more of a draw to spa goers. With this in mind, I've asked the experts at leading spas around the world to devise simple programs that you can do at home, based on the extensive menus on offer at their particular resorts. Take the time to road test the techniques for yourself. Once you find the method that's right for you, all it takes is regular practice and the results can be far reaching.

INSTANT STRESS-BUSTER TIPS

At work, meeting deadlines, or dealing with a difficult person, taking a deep breath and counting to ten could quite literally be what you need. During times of overload cultivate the art of stepping back to look at the "larger picture." To release stress in any situation, distance yourself mentally for a few minutes. Here, stress management expert Phyllis Pilgrim, based at Rancho La Puerta in Mexico, shares her quick-fix ways to help release the stress in your life.

1. Move physically out of the situation—go to a different room or go outside into the fresh air.
2. Inhale, stretching your arms up, then exhale and lower your arms. Repeat 5 to 10 times.
3. Take in a deep breath and count to ten as you exhale. With the exhalation, let problems and difficulties go.
4. Inhale positivity and solutions to your problems. Repeat 10 times.
5. Lower your shoulders and exhale. Roll your shoulders forward, then back. Repeat 10 times.
6. Smile as you inhale.
7. Exhale with strong exhalation sounds, blowing out your difficulties.
8. Breathe freely and stretch in any way that you like, as long as it feels comfortable.
9. Invite spaciousness and freedom into your consciousness.

An ancient Chinese exercise called *ki* can also help you to distance yourself psychologically from the immediate problem at hand and allow you to rediscover the larger perspective.

1. Stand with your feet slightly apart, knees bent, and hands over your abdomen.
2. Breathe rhythmically and tune in to your own energy (ki) through your breath.
3. Breathe in and lift your arms slowly to shoulder level—assess the situation.
4. As you exhale, step back with your right foot, bring your hands to your chest, elbows out sideways. Look at the larger picture.
5. Inhale, turn your palms out, then exhale and sweep your arms forward and sideways—clear away the clutter.
6. Inhale, bringing your hands in sideways to shoulders, palms out. Exhale, pressing your hands out sideways—create the space you are comfortable working in.
7. Inhale, stepping back, foot forward again, lowering your arms down to the side and up the front of your body—stepping back into the situation, seeing it from your new perspective.
8. Exhale, pressing your palms down to position your hands in front of your abdomen—return to the situation, calm and peaceful.
9. Repeat, but this time placing the left foot back rather than the right.

INSTANT CALMERS

There will be days when stress levels are soaring but you just can't squeeze in a calming session of yoga or meditation. The solution? Try one of these stress-reducing remedies.

Herbal helpers: There are a number of tried and true herbal remedies that help your body cope with stress more effectively and, in turn, will make you feel less harassed.

• Kava can be taken in supplement, infusion, or tincture form and will immediately give you a shot of calm.

• Panax ginseng helps the body to adapt to long-term stress but needs to be taken over a long period of time in order to be effective. Take in tincture or supplement form.

• Valerian root works well for those suffering from nervous tension and insomnia. Make an infusion of the root and take 1 cup up to three times a day.

• Chamomile and cowslip are also effective relaxants. Make an infusion with the petals and drink 1 cup two or three times a day.

Aromatherapy assets: Specific essential oils extracted from flowers and plants can help reduce the symptoms of stress overload and promote relaxation. Add them to your bath water or to a carrier oil and use to massage your temples, wrists, and hands for instant at-your-desk relief.

• *For tranquility:* Mix 2 drops petitgrain, 3 drops vetiver, and 3 drops clary sage.

• *For meditation:* Mix 2 drops cedarwood, 2 drops sandalwood, 2 drops frankincense, and 2 drops rose.

• *To soothe:* Mix 3 drops chamomile, 2 drops mandarin, and 2 drops ylang ylang.

• *To unwind:* Mix 2 drops geranium, 2 drops lavender, and 2 drops myrrh.

Flower power: Flower remedies such as those created by Dr Edward Bach and more recent versions like the Australian Bush Flower Essences, work on the emotions. Try these blends in your bath water when you are feeling worn to a frazzle.

• *To help overcome an office crisis:* Mix 2 drops each of white chestnut, walnut, vervain, olive, rock water, mustard, oak, and gentian.

• *To help prevent insomnia:* Mix 2 drops each of olive, rock rose, white chestnut, impatiens, and vervain.

• *When you are feeling down:* Mix 2 drops each of gentian, walnut, gorse, wild rose, sweet chestnut, and willow.

• *When you are feeling burnt out:* Mix 2 drops each of wild rose, walnut, mustard, oak, olive, elm, and gorse.

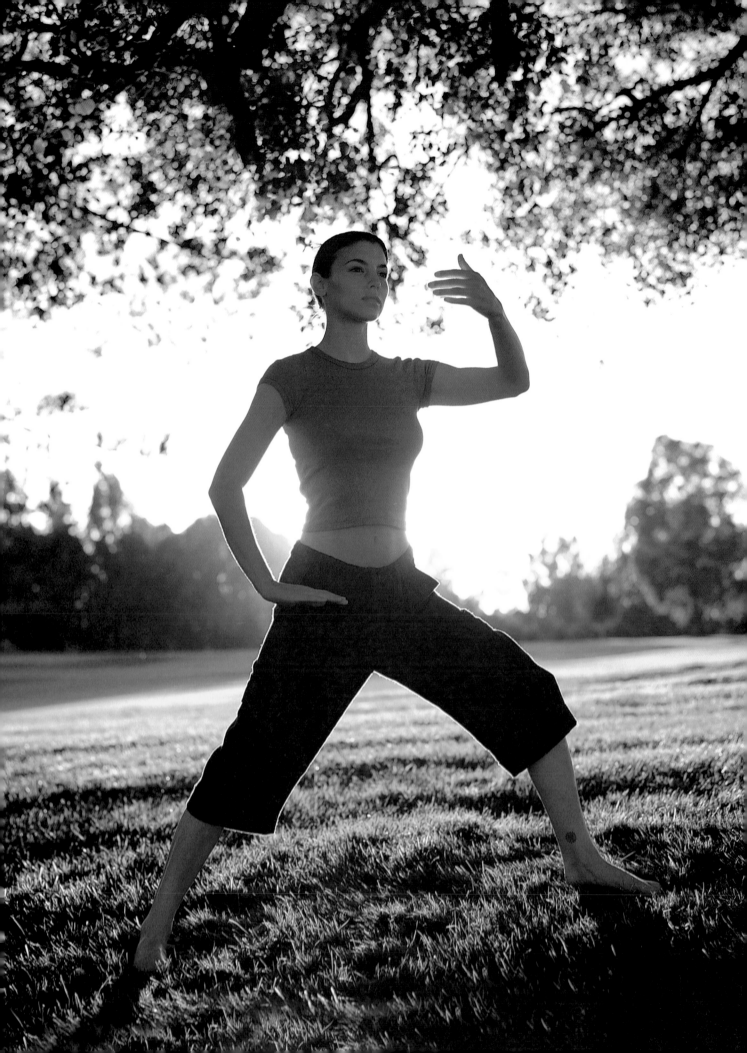

T'ai chi

It may originate in China, but t'ai chi has become a global form of movement therapy that is now almost as commonplace in Boston as it is in Beijing. Created in the thirteenth century by a Chinese Taoist monk, it is often described as an internal kung fu and aims to harness natural energy, both internally and externally. According to Taoist philosophy, chi (or life energy) has to flow freely through the body's energy channels or meridians to prevent disease and to establish well being through balance. When the energy is blocked, illness can set in, so it's crucial that these pathways remain open.

These days, t'ai chi forms a staple part of the relaxation and well being programs at many international spas. Not surprisingly, it has become as popular as yoga because of its potential health benefits if practiced regularly. Don't expect to be huffing and puffing if you take up t'ai chi. It's a peaceful, elegant form of movement that is incredibly meditative to do.

Made up of a series of graceful arm movements and leg postures, each movement symbolizes the process of harnessing the energy around us and drawing it into the body. The movements are performed in sequence that, at advanced levels, comprises 108 over a thirty-minute session. The sequence given here can but only touch on the full effect.

At spas such as the Ojai Valley Inn and Spa and the Golden Door, both in California, t'ai chi is one of the most popular relaxation techniques on the menu. There are many forms of t'ai chi from yang taijiquan to zenon wudang t'ai chi chuan, featured here.

The t'ai chi chuan sequence

This sequence has been adapted by Michael Jacques of T'ai Chi UK and represents the zenon wudang ta'i chi chuan system.

GUIDELINES

• Although t'ai chi chuan is extremely gentle and safe, it is wise to have a medical check-up before you start, especially if you suffer from a medical problem.

• Dress in loose, comfortable clothing. You don't need to wear shoes if training indoors. But if you are training outside, wear well-fitting shoes with cushioned, flexible soles and arch supports. Your toes should be able to move freely.

• T'ai chi chuan can be practiced at home, in a large room, in a park, or your garden. Ideally, you should join a class or find an instructor to learn the form correctly.

• You will get more benefits from t'ai chi chuan if you practice each day. Increase the amount of time you spend practicing as you become accustomed to the system.

• The more you practice, the better you will get and the more benefits you will gain. You will become mentally alert but relaxed, your mood will improve, and your confidence and self-esteem will be boosted.

• Regular practice has also been shown to improve the following ailments: diabetes mellitus (late onset), peripheral vascular disease, mild high blood pressure, asthma, and arthritis.

THE T'AI CHI MOVES

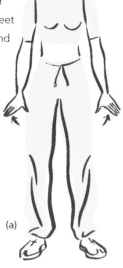

T'ai chi at rest
1. With your arms by your sides, palms down, and feet shoulder-width apart, bend your wrists, relax, and breathe normally (a).

(a)

T'ai chi ready style stance
2. Relax, with your hands down by your sides (b).

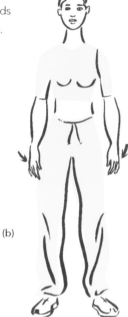

(b)

T'ai chi beginning style
3. Inhale and raise your arms in front of you to shoulder height.
4. Bend your arms and bring your hands to your shoulders.
5. Lower your arms.
6. Bend your knees softly.
7. Transfer all the weight to your right leg and then step forward on to your left heel.
8. Bring your left arm in front of you so that the palm faces the chest (c).
9. Bring your right arm in front of you so that the right palm faces the left palm. Also turn in your left foot and place it on the ground (d).
10. Transfer all your weight to your front leg by bending your left knee and straightening your right leg.

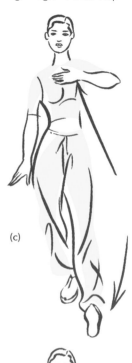

(c)

Seven stars style
11. Following on from the last position, reach out to the right with your right arm.
12. Keep your position, raise your right heel, and turn your body to the right.
13. Bring your left fingers in contact with your right wrist and step forwards on to your right heel.

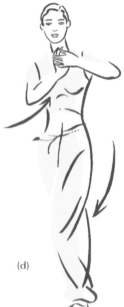

(d)

Yoga

Practiced in India for over three thousand years, yoga is increasingly popular and relevant to modern living. Yoga provides an effective antidote to the stresses that most of us suffer, combining spiritual, physical, and mental disciplines that aim to maintain the balance of mind, body, and spirit. To understand the scope of yoga and the effects produced, a six-day program has been designed at The Spa at Rajvilas, Jaipur, India. It includes basic poses, breathing exercises, and relaxation techniques. In addition there is a detoxifying program aimed at cleansing the systems of the body. At the end of the program, the aim is to:

• Have a rejuvenated and re-energized body.
• Get initiated into a logical philosophy of a healthier lifestyle.
• Develop self-discipline.
• Become aware of the self and the physical body.
• Become more aware of and responsive to the surroundings.
• Learn to relax.

(The program is not intended for those who suffer from medical problems. In such cases, seek the advice of an experienced teacher/doctor.)

The program's benefits are optimized if it is coupled with detoxifying changes in the diet. Abstain from alcohol, tobacco, tea, coffee, meat and animal products, onions, garlic, and carbonated drinks. These produce toxins, which may inhibit the efficient functioning of the body's systems. As a yogic lifestyle is closely associated to ayurveda, the intake of these foods, which act as stimulants producing tamasic (gross) effects in the body, must be abstained from.

Mild withdrawal symptoms such as headache, nausea, and diarrhea may be experienced. These symptoms also indicate that detoxification is taking place within your bodily system. All the same, if any of the symptoms persist for more than two days, please consult an experienced teacher/doctor. The postures on the following pages are chosen because they help to achieve equilibrium for both the physical body and the bio-energies at a subtler level. They may help in stopping or reducing quite considerably the use of caffeine, nicotine, and alcohol. The awareness of breathing reduces stress levels.

The yogic rejuvenation

GUIDELINES

• It is advisable while following the program to have light meals with an increased intake of water, milk, juices, and fresh vegetables and fruits. There should be at least four to five hours between a meal and the yoga session.
• Practice yoga in a clean, quiet, well-ventilated environment. Though the preference of time differs with each of us, practice whenever you are not in a hurry.
• Clothing should be light and comfortable and should not hinder the movements of your body.
• You will need two blankets and one non-slip mattress to perform these postures.
• A light snack of milk with fruits is suggested an hour after the end of the session.

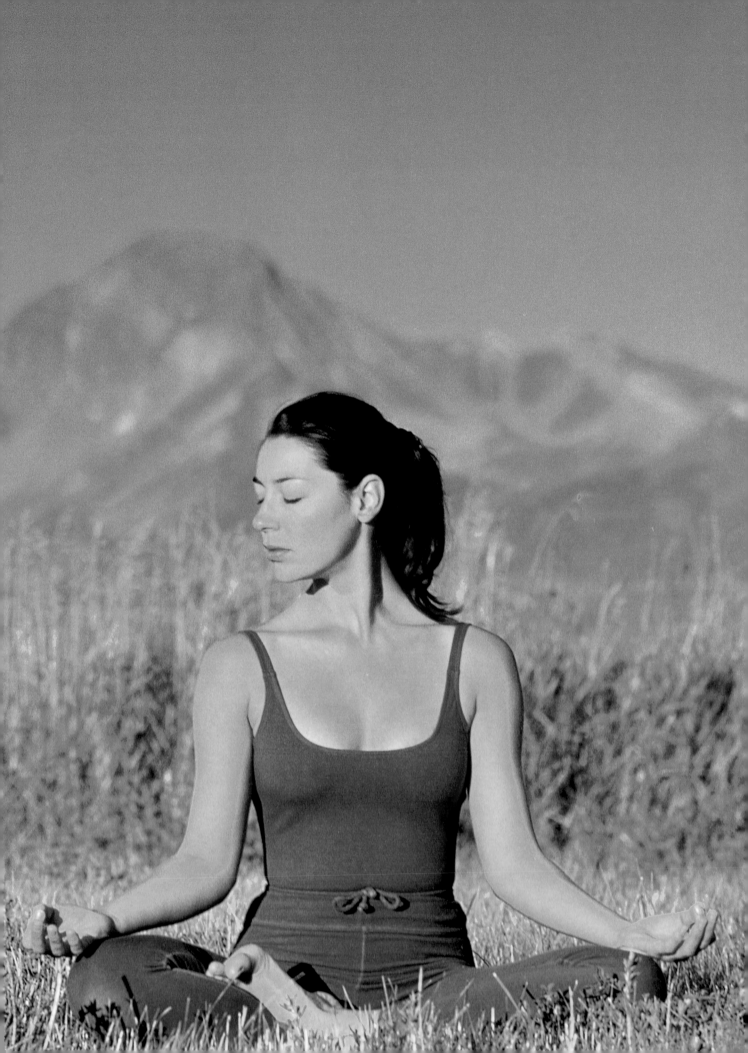

The yogic rejuvenation program

from The Spa at Rajvilas, Jaipur, India

DAY 1

Breathing check (general)

Lie down on your back as comfortably as possible, leaving your whole body relaxed. Close your eyes and become aware of your breathing. After 2 to 3 minutes, put your right hand on your stomach. Now observe the movement of the hand. With each inhalation your hand should rise and with each exhalation, it should fall.

Sukhasana (easy pose)

This pose is performed by sitting cross-legged and with your eyes open. Sit on a folded blanket, with your legs crossed over the mattress and at the shins. Your spine and the neck are slightly extended; the shoulders slightly pulled back. Your body weight is evenly supported; breathing is slow, smooth, and effortless (a). Become aware of your physical body and your surroundings. Hold the pose for 2 to 3 minutes. Slowly straighten your legs and relax for a moment; re-cross, changing the position of the legs. Hold for 2 to 3 minutes. Repeat the whole set once.

(a)

Vajrasana (rock pose)

Perform this movement by kneeling down with your knees kept together and sitting, evenly balancing your body between the calves and the heels. Your spine and neck are kept straight and the shoulders are even. Keep the eyes open and become aware of your body and also your surroundings. Breathe slowly and smoothly. Hold for 2 to 3 minutes. Repeat once after relaxing the legs for a minute.

Bhadrasna (rock pose variant)

Sit in the rock pose as performed before but this time slowly cross your hands behind your back, at the lower back level; keep your eyes open. Bend your neck forwards and fix your gaze between the knees at an imaginary point. Feel the expansion of your chest and shoulders with each inhalation. Hold for 2 to 3 minutes. Repeat once after resting the legs for 1 minute.

Caution: In case of neck pain or problems, do not bend your neck. Keep it straight and gaze at an imaginary point at eye level.

Makarasana (crocodile pose)

Lie flat on your stomach on a mattress with your arms stretched above your head and with your chin on the mattress; give a slight stretch to the body, keeping the big toes together. Fix your gaze between your hands and continue to hold for 2 to 3 minutes.

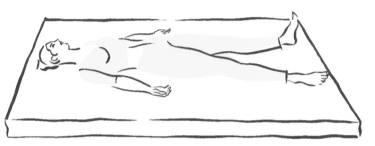

(b)

Shavasana (corpse pose)

Slowly turn over to lie down on your back, with your eyes closed. Let your whole body's weight be on the mattress. Slowly become aware of your body. Let your legs, trunk, shoulders, arms, and neck become loose (b). Become aware of your breathing; inhale slowly and smoothly and exhale the same way. Observe the rise and the fall of your stomach. Relax in this position for 10 to 12 minutes. Then get up slowly.

DAY 2

Tadasana (palm tree pose)

This is a static pose in which you stand with your big toes and ankles together. Your spine and neck are extended slightly and shoulders slightly pulled back. Let your arms hang loose at your sides. The body is kept balanced on your feet while maintaining the whole posture evenly. Fix your gaze at an imaginary point straight ahead. Breathe slowly and smoothly. Maintain this pose for 30 to 60 seconds and repeat twice.

Caution: Do not jump into the pose and do not overextend your knees.

Vriksasana (the tree pose)

Stand in tadasana. Slowly raise your left leg sideways, bend it at the knee and position the foot on the top of your inner left thigh. Slowly raise your arms and stretch them above the head joining the palms (c). Fix your gaze at an imaginary point straight ahead. Breathe slowly and smoothly. Maintain for 30 to 60 seconds. Repeat, alternating the legs. Repeat the set.

Caution: Do not jump into the pose and do not overbalance on one foot; keep it firmly on the floor. Do not overextend your knees.

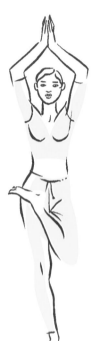

(c)

Ashwathasana (the peepul tree pose)

Stand in tadasana and raise your left arm straight above your head and the right one towards the side, palm downwards. Gradually stretch your right leg backwards without bending the knee and maintain the pose for 30 to 60 seconds. Repeat, alternating the position of your hands and legs. Repeat the set.

Caution: Do not jump into the pose and do not overbalance on one foot; keep it firmly on the floor. Do not overextend your knees.

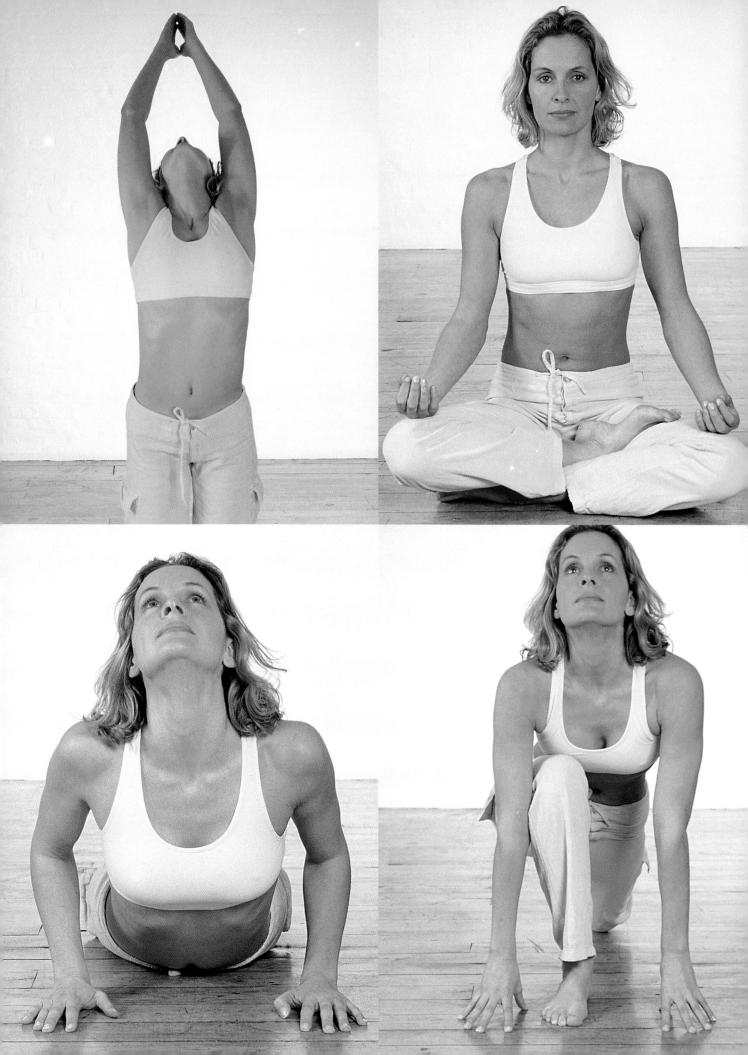

Veerasana (hero's pose)

Stand in tadasana and stretch your right leg backwards. Rest the right knee on the floor so that the left leg is bent at the knee. Raise your arms parallel to your shoulders in front of your body and clench the fists. Slowly straighten your right leg so that the weight is on the left leg. Extend the left arm and flex the right one so that your elbow touches your waist. Hold for 60 to 90 seconds. Repeat, alternating the position of the legs and the arms. Repeat the set.

Shavasana (corpse pose)

Slowly turn over to lie down on your back, with your eyes closed. Let your whole body's weight be on the mattress. Slowly become aware of your body. Let your legs, trunk, shoulders, arms, and neck become loose. Become aware of your breathing; inhale slowly and smoothly and exhale the same way. Observe the rise and the fall of your stomach. Relax in this position for 10 to 12 minutes. Then get up slowly.

DAY 3

Repeat the poses done on Days 1 and 2 except for shavasana, a longer version of which is given below to finish your yoga exercises for Day 3.

On Day 3 for all the seated poses, keep your eyes closed; breathe as in shavasana, slowly and smoothly, and visualize that your body is being enveloped in a warm aura of energy. Repeat each pose three times, holding each for 2 to 3 minutes.

For all the standing poses, keep your eyes open; breathe as in shavasana; keep your gaze fixed and visualize your body as it appears in the pose. Feel the energies of the body getting balanced and flowing throughout the body.

Repeat all poses three times, holding each between 30 and 90 seconds.

Shavasana (corpse pose)

Lie down on your back, with your eyes closed. Let your whole body's weight be on the mattress. Slowly become aware of your body. Let your legs, trunk, shoulders, arms, and neck become loose. Become aware of your breathing; inhale slowly and smoothly and exhale the same way. Observe the rise and the fall of your stomach. Inhale normally and exhale smoothly and slowly without straining yourself; let the exhalation be longer than the inhalation. Relax and keep the breathing rhythm for 5 to 6 minutes. Stay in the shavasana for 10 to 12 minutes.

THE LONG-TERM BENEFITS OF YOGA

• Regular practice of yoga has been shown to improve oxygen supply to the blood, thereby benefiting the circulation.

• Since yoga focuses on carefully balanced stretches and postures, there tends to be less risk of joint problems.

• Deeper breathing helps to reduce conditions such as asthma, and can reduce the likelihood of panic attacks and hyperventilation.

• Conditions such as constipation are also alleviated because yogic breathing and postures help stimulate the digestive system.

• Yoga helps to reduce blood pressure, stress-related headaches, and back pain caused by tension and poor posture.

Aikido

According to Daintree spa's resident ki aikido specialist, Roby Kessler, regular practice of these Japanese exercises helps to bring harmony and vitality to our lives. Not only do they promote physical and mental health in the individual, but they also influence our daily interactions with others. "Ki is the universal energy that can be directed through the mind, which then affects the body. You may have heard the saying: Where the mind goes the body will follow," says Kessler.

Ki development was founded in the early twentieth century by Morihei Ueshiba. Koichi Tonei, who was Ueshiba's chief instructor, went on to espouse the fundamental ki aikido principles:

1. Ki is extending.
2. Know your opponent's mind.
3. Respect your opponent's ki.
4. Put yourself in your opponent's place.
5. Lead with confidence.

A beginner's ki aikido course

from Daintree Eco-Lodge and Spa, Queensland, Australia

Supporting the Daintree Eco Lodge philosophy that mind/body connection influences good health, staff and guests are invited to participate in morning ki aikido sessions. Like t'ai chi and yoga, aikido is best learnt from a qualified instructor. However, Roby Kessler has devised a beginner's course that you can practice at home.

GUIDELINES

• The following stretching exercises serve to unify the mind and body when in motion.
• Perform the movements in a fluid and comfortable manner.
• Remember to keep your mind and body unified by following any one of the following principles: keep centered; relax completely; keep your weight underside (where the weight naturally falls), and extend ki–do what you do with 100 percent focus.
• Work in an open space, preferably at a comfortable room temperature.
• Wear loose, warm clothing.
• Put on some music of your choice, preferably soft with a slight beat.

TOITSU-TAISO (COORDINATION EXERCISES)

Trunk twist
Stand with your feet apart and with a shoulder-width distance between them. Twist the trunk from side to side by swinging the arms (a).
Left: count 1-2; Right: count 3-4;
Left: count 5-6; Right: count 7-8.
Perform twice.

(a)

Bend the trunk to the side

Left: count 1-2; Right: count 3-4; Left: count 5-6;
Right: count 7-8.
Perform twice.

Bend backward and forward (knees bent)

Backward: count 1-2; Forward:
count 3-4; Backward: count 5-6;
Forward: count 7-8. Perform twice
(b and c).

(b)

(c)

Shoulder blade exercise

Bend your arms in front of you and then raise
your elbows so that they are parallel with the
floor, then gently push left shoulder back, then
right shoulder back twice.
Left: count 1-2; Right: count 3-4; Left: count 5-6;
Right: count 7-8.
Perform twice.

Neck stretches

Bend your neck from left to right, with each ear moving toward
the corresponding shoulder blade. Repeat. Then carefully bend
the neck from front to back in a controlled manner. Repeat.
Left: count 1-2; Right: count 3-4; Left: count 5-6; Right: count
7-8. Forward: count 1-2; Backward: count 3-4; Forward: count 5-
6; Right: Backward 7-8.

Arm swings 1

Standing upright with feet slightly apart, swing one arm
(forward swing only) at a time.
Left arm: count 1-2-3-4; Right arm: count 5-6-7-8.
Perform twice.

Arm swings 2

Swing both arms (d).
Forward: count 1-2-3-4;
Backward: count 5-6-7-8.
Perform twice.

Arm swings 3

Now swing both arms while
gently bending the knees.
Forward: count 1-2-3-4;
Backward: count 5-6-7-8.
Perform twice.

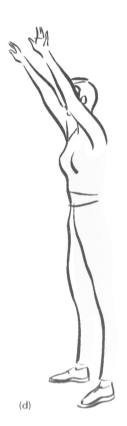

(d)

Meditation

Once upon a time, we Westerners viewed meditation with scepticism. It was practiced by Eastern gurus who spent their lives in isolation in search of Nirvana and enlightenment or adopted by neo-hippies as a legal way of "getting high." How times have changed. Now considered by many as commonplace as aromatherapy, some forms of meditation such as transcendental meditation are even recommended by doctors as an effective solution for stress-related conditions. At health spas in the east and west, you are just as likely to find meditation on the menu as you are aerobic and stretch classes. The reason? Regular practice of meditation techniques has been proven to lower blood pressure, lessen the risk of developing certain diseases, including cancer, and to generally boost the immune system. Not only that, meditation is a sure-fire way of allowing us to tune in to our natural state of tranquility.

The Expanding Light yoga and meditation retreat was founded over twenty-seven years ago in the Sierra Nevada foothills of northern California. Famed for their yoga and meditation workshops, devotees travel from around the world to learn the art of tranquility in this truly peaceful retreat. Based on the universal teachings of the great Indian master, Paramhansa Yogananda, author of the spiritual classic *Autobiography of a Yogi*, the workshops recognize that everyone's path is unique, that true spiritual growth should benefit every aspect of your life, and that it comes from inner experience, not blind belief. The Expanding Light exists to support guests in their search.

So exactly what does meditation do for us? "Meditation offers a wide variety of real benefits that have a deep-reaching impact on our lives," explains Marilyn Carr, The Expanding Light's director. "The meditator experiences greater peace, calmness, and joy as the mind quiets and the heart expands. All areas of life–work, relationships and health–begin miraculously to change as the true Self comes home to itself."

With regular practice, problems are solved more easily and work done more quickly because energies are focused. You can also act calmly in the face of difficult situations rather than reacting out of frustration and concentrate more deeply. "Everything in life will, in time, look and feel different because it will be infused with that peace and joy that is our true nature," adds Carr.

"It is not, as so many people assume it to be, a process of 'thinking things over.' Rather, it is making the mind completely receptive to reality. It is stilling the thought-processes–those restless ripples that bob on the surface of the mind–so that truth, like the moon, may be clearly reflected there. It is listening to God, to Universal Reality, for a change, instead of doing all the talking and 'computing' oneself," explains Carr.

THE BENEFITS OF MEDITATION

• Meditation significantly controls high blood pressure at levels comparable to widely used prescription drugs, and without the side effects.

• Chronic pain can be reduced by more than 50 percent.

• 75 percent of long-term insomniacs who are trained in meditation find that they can fall asleep within twenty minutes of going to bed.

• Meditation decreases oxygen consumption, heart rate, respiratory rate, and blood pressure, and increases the intensity of brain waves–the opposite of the physiological changes that occur during the stress response.

• Meditators have been shown to be less anxious and neurotic, more spontaneous, independent, self-confident, empathetic, and less fearful of death.

HOW TO PRACTICE MEDITATION

At The Expanding Light, meditation goes hand in hand with hatha yoga. For the best results, begin with perhaps half an hour of yoga postures or asanas and 15 minutes of meditation and increase the practices gradually as your mind and body are ready to do so. Instructions and guidelines are given here.

The ideal way to learn yoga and meditation would be on retreat from an experienced practitioner. This has many advantages, one being that you leave your daily concerns and tasks behind and can turn all of your attention to the incorporation of new practices into your life while being at a peaceful site that carries a vibration to support this new learning. It is important to carefully select such a place, one that feels right for you. The next best scenario would be to attend a local meditation and yoga workshop or course as these practices are most easily demonstrated visually by someone you can relate to personally. Then, as with the retreat option, you can incorporate the practices into your home routine.

If none of the above is possible in the near future, there's no need to wait. The instructions given on the following pages can get you started on a powerful and transformative home practice. But read the following advice first.

GETTING COMFORTABLE FOR A SITTING MEDITATION

Before starting your meditation there are a few things that you can do to help the smooth flowing of your session.

Perform some yoga postures and energizing exercises: Yoga postures are a wonderful way to get the energy flowing. Or use other gentle exercises of your choice which calm, rather than excite, the nervous system.

Say a prayer: Always ask for guidance. Say a prayer mentally or out loud in whatever form feels comfortable to you. Don't forget this important step when practicing meditation.

Do some chanting: If you don't play a musical instrument, have a chanting tape to sing along with, either out loud or mentally. Chanting opens the heart, an important ingredient for deep meditation.

Sit comfortably: One of the most important aspects of a sitting meditation is to be able to sit comfortably, without suffering an aching back or legs that hurt or are falling asleep. If you are in pain or great discomfort, the only thing you will be meditating on is that! The options for sitting are in a chair, on a meditation bench, or on a pillow on the floor. Most Westerners are not trained from birth to sit comfortably on a hard floor. So a chair is probably best for most people, beginners or otherwise, and many very great meditators with many years experience use a chair or stool for their meditations. It is not a sign of lack of meditative ability if you are unable to sit in the lotus posture or any other position.

Get a fairly straight-backed chair and sit forward in the chair so that both feet are flat on the floor. If your feet do not touch the floor, get a shorter chair or place a pillow or two under your feet to raise them so that your thighs are parallel to the floor. Do not lean against the back of the chair. The idea is to sit with an unsupported and upright spine. However, if you are not used to sitting this way, or if you have weak neck/back muscles or injuries in these areas, there are ways

PRACTICAL HINTS FOR MEDITATION

Schedule: Set aside the same time or times each day for your meditation. Recommended times are dawn (just after waking up), twilight, noon, and midnight. Another is in the evening, just before bedtime. It is always best to meditate on an empty stomach (2 to 3 hours after meals).

Location: Set aside a room, or small part of a room, just for meditation. Try to find as quiet a spot as possible or, if this is difficult, try using comfortable foam earplugs or headphones to block out noise. Be sure the room is not stuffy and that it is a bit on the cool side. Have a place to sit, and a small, simple altar or focal point, with pictures, flowers, and candles on it. You will find that the vibrations of meditation build here. If possible, face east while meditating. Yogis say that there are certain natural currents that flow east to west, and these help you meditate better.

Use a blanket or two: Many yogis recommend sitting on a wool rug, blanket, or piece of silk. Also as the place you are meditating in should be a little on the cool side with, if possible, a source of fresh air, another blanket or warm meditation shawl should be handy to wrap up in. The body does cool down when you sit still for a while, so a wrap is often important to maintain an even body temperature during your meditation session. Get yourself comfortable, but stay awake and ready!

Say a little prayer: Upon beginning your meditation, say a prayer either out loud, or inwardly, to God or a higher power, to guide and help you. It is also helpful to do some chanting, if you can (using a cassette tape of chants is very nice–sing along with it!).

Meditate with joy and devotion: Don't wait to be made joyful, be joyful first yourself! Meditation simply helps you remember, on deepening levels of awareness, who and what you really are.

to overcome this challenge. Get a firm pillow and put it between your back and the back of the chair. The feeling you want is that of support, but not leaning into it. Move the pillow around until you achieve this feeling. If you want to place a pillow in the seat of the chair, to cushion a surface that is too hard, that is fine.

Meditate for short periods of time in the beginning and work up to longer amounts of time. In this way, your back muscles will gradually strengthen. Yoga stretches and other such exercises also strengthen your back muscles with time and regular practice. Do not set unrealistic goals for yourself. It is better to meditate for 5 to 15 minutes and be consistent about it, and then increase your time as you can. One longer meditation each week is very helpful.

Meditation benches are a wonderful invention for making the legs feel comfortable and un-pressured and keeping the spine upright. Finding the right size and height is important. Padding on the seat often helps. Adding small pillows under the knees or ankles might also make you more comfortable. If you have never tried a bench, please be sure to experiment with one. Some people are more comfortable sitting cross-legged on a pillow. You can buy crescent-shaped or round, plump pillows, which are designed to help with this position.

So experiment. Have a chair, lots of pillows, a bench, and whatever else you want to try at hand. When one position becomes tiresome, calmly switch to another. Eventually you will find the best position for your body type. Remember that everybody's body is different. You should feel relatively relaxed once you have finished meditating but sitting on the wrong chair or without sufficient pillows will make this state more difficult to achieve.

The Hong-Sau technique of meditation

from The Expanding Light, California

The breath and mind react intimately to each other. The breath instantly responds to different mental and emotional states. As the breath flows, so flows the mind. By concentrating on the breath, the mind becomes calmer. This is the Hong-Sau technique of concentration and meditation as taught by Paramhansa Yogananda and also by his disciple Swami Kriyananda, the founder and spiritual director of The Expanding Light, and it is this technique that is described here.

1. Energization, prayer, and chanting are suggested before meditation, but Hong-Sau actually may be done at any time and in any place. If you have time, exercise a little before meditation. Yoga postures are excellent and, of course, Yogananda's energization exercises are highly recommended. Remember that the exercises you do before meditation should calm, not excite, the nervous system.

2. Inhale and tense the whole body. Exhale and relax. Repeat three times. Then, inhale slowly to a count of 6 to 10; hold the breath to that same count; exhale to that count and immediately inhale again to the same count. Repeat 6 to 10 times. Please remember that these are preliminary breathing exercises, not the technique itself.

3. Now, without counting or tension, take a long, slow, deep breath. When the breath begins to flow again, begin to observe its movement, without any attempt to control it. Notice the place at which you can observe the breath in your body whether in the lungs, in the nostrils, or sinuses. Be an impartial observer, not caring whether it flows in or out or remains stationary. Simply remain attentive to whatever the breath does by itself, naturally. Moving the forefinger of the right hand in for inhalation and out for exhalation may help you to tune into your breathing.

4. Follow the inhalation with the mantra Hong (pronounced to rhyme with song) and the exhalation with the mantra Sau (pronounced like saw). Repeat the mantra mentally only. Be careful not to move the lips or tongue. Hong-Sau is a Sanskrit mantra meaning "I am He" or "I am Spirit."

5. As your practice deepens, begin to enjoy the pauses between the inhalations and the exhalations, when the breath is not flowing. Do not actively hold the breath in or out. As many times as your mind wanders away from Hong-Sau, bring it gently back to the technique.

6. After your period of practice of this technique (5 to 10 minutes is fine for beginners, gradually increasing the time as you go), inhale and exhale three times, and then leave the breath out for as long as is comfortable for you. Then begin breathing normally once again.

7. Throughout the practice, keep your eyes closed and looking upward towards the point between the eyebrows; don't strain your eyes–let them relax!

8. After completing your practice of Hong-Sau, be sure to sit in silence and stillness for at least as long as you practiced the technique. During this time, practice devotion, inward chanting, visualization, or prayer. Hold your body still and be very silent and relaxed, yet aware.

The powerful meditation/concentration technique of Hong-Sau may bring you ever closer to your highest potential.

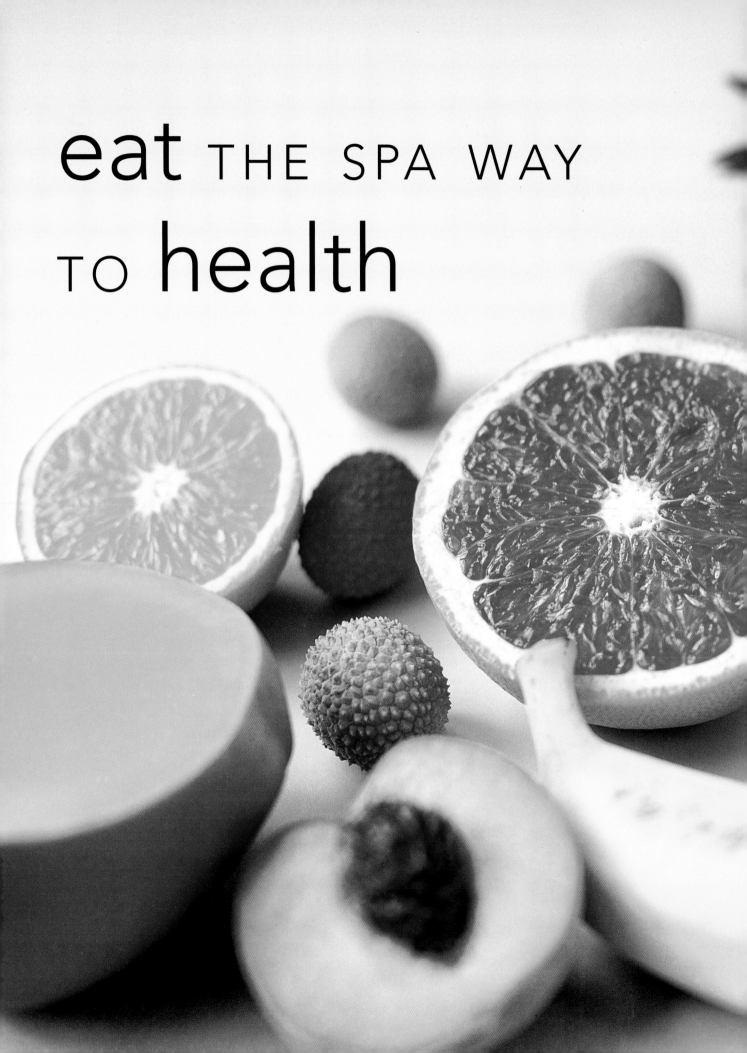

eat THE SPA WAY
TO health

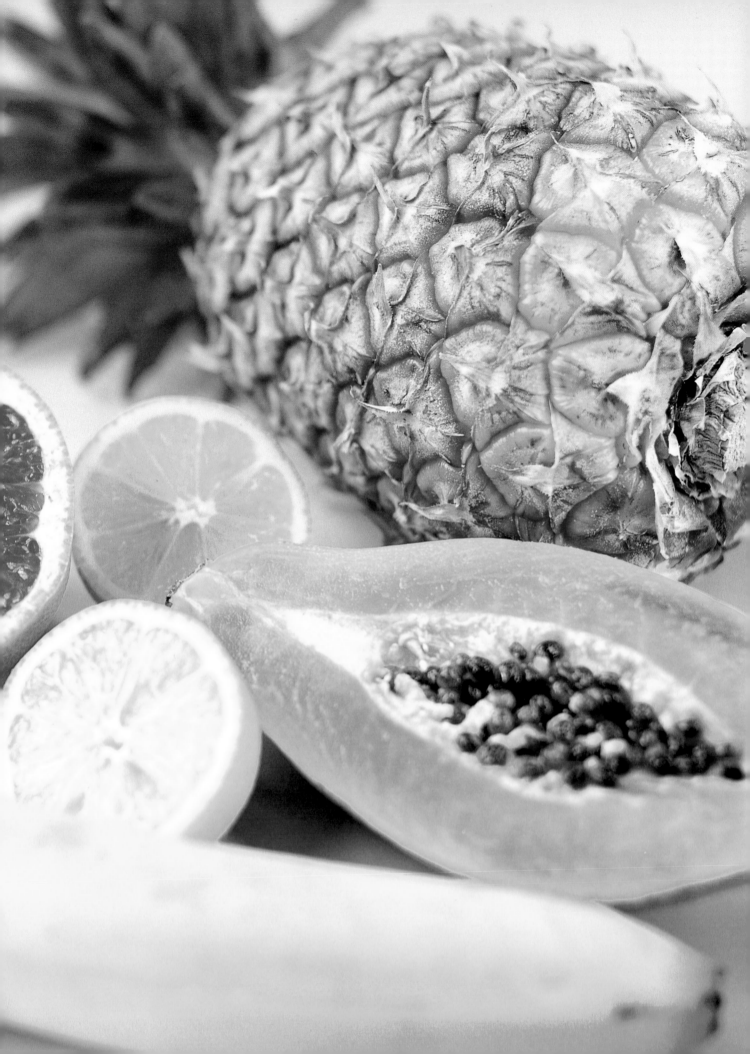

The spa food philosophy

When it comes to eating well, nobody's perfect. Even nutritionists and health gurus more than occasionally forget to practice what they preach, swigging the odd glass of champagne and skipping meals from time to time. No one wants to be dictated to when it comes to what we eat but we all know that apart from the incredibly virtuous, our diets could be better. As well as the obvious fact that sometimes "bad" things are too good to resist, the main reason that most of us go off the wagon—once in a while or perpetually—comes down to lifestyle. It's all too easy when we are feeling fractious and fatigued to forget about health food and load up on junk food.

Be it late-night take-out or fast food grabbed on the run, we are constantly depriving ourselves of freshly prepared meals that are nutrient-rich, not to mention delicious. While we can't always book in to a spa to re-educate our palette and detoxify our bodies, we can benefit from culinary spa know-how at home. I've gathered some of the best recipes from premier spas around the world so that you can create your own home-spa food program. You can use it as a once-in-a-while detox and to boost vital nutrients or you might be completely converted and never return to convenience and fast food again.

The philosophy behind spa food is simple, not to mention universal. It is designed to feed your body on all levels, with colors and textures that are visually appealing and tastes and aromas that satisfy, stimulate, and cleanse. Contrary to popular belief, the food served up at modern spas and health resorts does not consist of a few meager bean sprouts or a bowl of mushy gruel,

as some of my non-spa-going friends seem to think. It can be as delicious and sophisticated as anything you might find on any haute cuisine menu anywhere in the world. First-class chefs are employed to create tantalizing food that also has a healthy spin. It's obvious that low fat, salt, and sugar is the order of the day—but that doesn't mean the food tastes bland. Far from it, as I hope you will find out from first-hand experience.

SIMPLE GUIDELINES FOR BALANCE

The secret to eating healthfully—no surprises here –is balance. Whether you are cooking at home, dining out, or choosing take-out, here are a few tips that I have gathered from the experts at Canyon Ranch in Arizona.

Fruits and vegetables: Every meal should include fruits or vegetables, and preferably both. If you make these foods the central component of a meal, you won't overlook them. Research has shown that a diet that is rich in fruits and vegetables is rich in disease-fighting nutrients such as antioxidants and phytochemicals. Try to include five to nine servings from this food group every day by including them in soups, salads, sandwich filings, stir-fries, and juices.

Carbohydrate-rich foods: This category includes beans, soybeans, peas, corn, potatoes, brown and wild rice, and grains including barley and millet, and breads and pasta made from any of these grains. Being rich in carbohydrates and fiber, they also include some protein. Make sure you get plenty of variety and don't just stick with white breads and pasta. Always stick to moderately sized portions.

Protein-rich foods: Fish, poultry, soy foods, beans, eggs, low-fat dairy foods, nuts, seeds, and lean meat are in this category. These foods are the most concentrated sources of protein and through including them in a meal you will help to satisfy hunger and sustain energy levels.

Fat: At Canyon Ranch and many other spas, it is suggested that about 20 percent of total calorie intake comes from fat. You may need to tailor this to your own preferences and health conditions. It means that you should be eating about 25 to 40 grams of fat a day from the healthiest sources, which include extra virgin olive oil, olives, nuts, seeds, avocados, and fatty fish like salmon and tuna. It is wise to limit hydrogenated fat as much as possible, usually found in margarine, cookies, and other processed food. Don't completely cut it out, unless your doctor advises you to do so.

Fiber: Low-fat diets can be low in fiber because they are centered around white flour products like bagels and pasta. You should get 25 to 40 grams of dietary fiber each day in the form of bran cereal, whole grains, beans, fruits, and vegetables. Not only does fiber help to maintain blood sugar levels, it lowers cholesterol levels and also helps to keep the digestive system in peak condition. New research has also suggested that fiber influences hormone levels and affects the immune system.

Salt and sugar: Try to keep salt intake to a minimum, particularly if you suffer from high blood pressure. If you do use salt, choose natural sea salt. As for sugar, most spas try to limit the use of refined sugar, opting instead for molasses, honey, fruit juice concentrate, and fructose.

Water: Most nutritionists advocate drinking at least eight glasses a day. The general consensus is that water is essential to dilute the waste materials excreted by the body. This ensures that kidneys are not over-worked and also prevents dehydration. Coffee and tea are not water substitutes. In fact, caffeinated beverages are diuretics and only serve to further dehydrate your body. If you are addicted to hot drinks, swap to herbal tisanes, or try a little lemon juice and honey in hot water as a tea or coffee replacement.

SPA COOKING TIPS
• Use plenty of herbs and spices. As they contain practically no calories, they can be used liberally to flavor foods. Sprinkle them on salads and in soups and casseroles to replace salt and compensate for fat.
• Use non-stick pots and pans. Cut down on your use of oil by cooking everything from fish, poultry, and pancakes in non-stick cookware.
• Cook or roast at a low temperature for a longer period of time. Using slow-cookers or roasting in an oven at a very low temperature helps flavors to blend and creates a rich-tasting dish with little or no fat.

Breakfast

Most nutritionists consider that breakfast is the most important meal of the day, yet many of us tend to skip it because we're in too much of a hurry. Make an effort to include a satisfying, nutritious breakfast each day, even if it's only for one week once a month. You don't need to spend hours preparing it–a simple feast of fresh fruit and yogurt, wholegrain bread, and an herbal tea will set you up for the day ahead.

Grilled banana with cashew nuts and honey served with fresh fruit

from the Nusa Dua Spa, Bali, Indonesia
Makes 4 servings

4 bananas
¼ cup honey
¼ cup chopped cashew nuts
½ cup plain yogurt
¼ cup orange juice
2 tsp dextrose
4 sticks lemon grass or wooden kebab sticks
½ cup chopped papaya
½ cup chopped watermelon
¼ cup grapefruit segments

1. Slice the bananas in half and grill until they are a little soft.
2. Brush the grilled bananas with honey and sprinkle with the chopped cashew nuts.
3. Grill again until golden brown.
4. Combine the yogurt, orange juice, and dextrose. Then arrange the fresh fruit on the plates and pour the yogurt-orange mix around the edge.
5. Skewer the bananas on a lemon grass or wooden stick, pile on top of the fruit and serve.

Granola

from Rancho La Puerta, Baja California, Mexico
Makes 6 servings

3 cups old-fashioned rolled oats
½ cup chopped almonds
½ cup sunflower seeds
¼ cup wholewheat flour
¼ cup oat bran
1 tbsp ground cinnamon
¾ tsp ground ginger
1 tsp cardamom
¾ cup honey
½ cup unsweetened, unfiltered apple juice
2 tbsp vanilla extract
2 tsp canola oil
2 tsp grated orange zest
2 tbsp fresh orange juice (optional)

1. Preheat the oven to 250°F. Lightly coat a baking sheet with vegetable oil spray.
2. In a large mixing bowl, combine the rolled oats, almonds, seeds, flour, oat bran, cinnamon, ginger, and cardamom.
3. In another bowl, whisk together the honey, apple juice, vanilla, and oil until the honey is thoroughly incorporated. Add the orange zest and the orange juice, if desired.
4. Pour the wet ingredients over the dry ingredients and mix well. Spread the granola evenly over the baking sheet and bake for 1½ hours, checking every 15 minutes. When the granola starts to brown, stir gently with a spatula. Be sure that the outside edges do not burn. When golden and dry, scrape on to a plate or a cool baking sheet and set aside to cool. Store in an airtight container until ready to use.

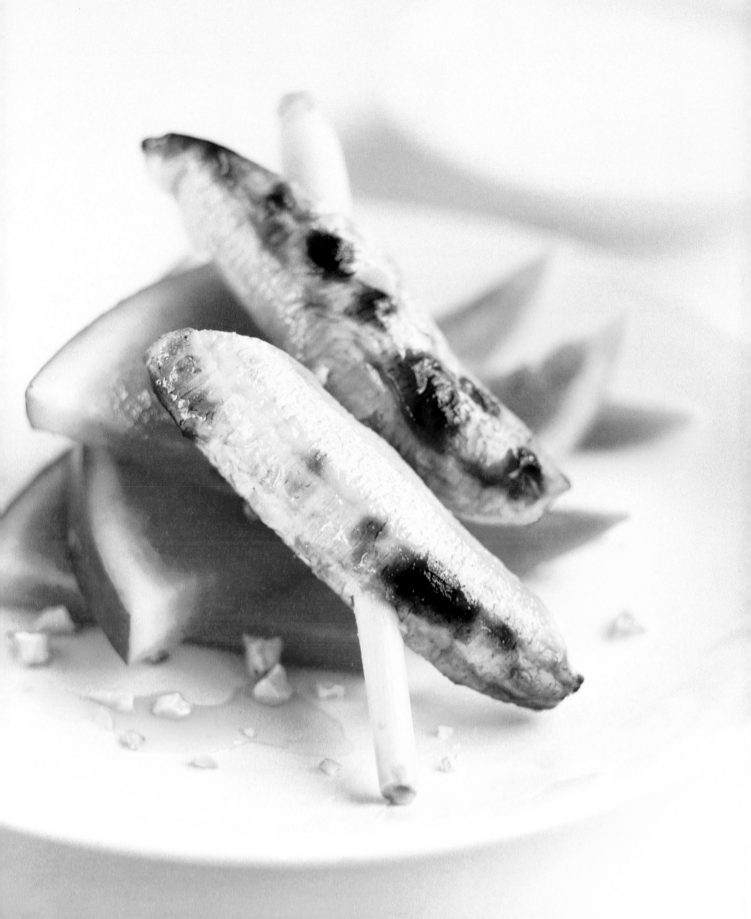

Alpine muesli

from Canyon Ranch, Arizona

Makes 8 servings

½ cup uncooked quick porridge oats
1 cup skim milk
½ cup plain non- or low-fat yogurt
1 cup orange juice
⅓ cup ground hazelnuts
¼ cup fructose or honey
1 lb apples, grated
1 lb freshly chopped fruit such as peach, apricot, and melon

1. In a large bowl, combine the oats, skim milk, and yogurt. Let it stand for 5 minutes to soften the oats.
2. Add the orange juice, ground nuts, and fructose or honey. Stir thoroughly.
3. Grate the apple and stir into the mixture to prevent the apple from browning. Stir in the chopped fruit. Serve chilled.

Oatmeal muesli bars

from Forest Mere Health Farm, Hampshire, UK

Makes 30 muesli bars

4 cups all-purpose flour
6 cups oats
2½ tsp baking powder
3 cups granulated sugar
1 lb margarine
5 tbsp honey
1 cup natural yogurt

1. Put the flour, oats, and baking powder into a mixing bowl.
2. Heat the sugar, margarine, and honey together, very gently.
3. When all the ingredients are melted together pour on to the oats and flour, adding the yogurt, and mix well until combined.
4. Add the flavorings (see below) and pour into a tray lined with parchment paper and spread evenly.
5 Bake at 300°F for 15 to 20 minutes.

IDEAS FOR FLAVORINGS

Apple and date: Put 1½ cups of dried apple and ½ cup of dried stoned dates into a food processor and pulse until roughly chopped. Add to the muesli mix before spreading on the baking tray.

Apricot and sunflower seed: Put 2 cups of dried apricots in a food processor and pulse until roughly chopped, then add 1 cup of sunflower seeds and add to the muesli mix as above.

Currant and pumpkin seed: Add 2 cups of currants and 1 cup of pumpkin seeds to the muesli mix.

Prune and almond: Add 2 cups of pitted prunes and 1½ cups of flaked almonds to the mix.

Oatmeal

from the Golden Door, California

Makes 4 servings

"Victoria Reynoso, who is in charge of breakfast at The Golden Door, revealed her secret for delicious oatmeal. Patience and a very low flame are their own reward. For the best flavor and texture, serve the oatmeal as soon as it thickens," says Michel Stroot, executive chef of the Golden Door.

1 cup old-fashioned rolled oats
¼ tsp salt (optional)
¼ tsp ground cinnamon
1 red or green apple, peeled, cored, and grated
8 tsp honey
¼ cup raisins or currants

1. In a medium sized saucepan, bring 2 cups of water to the boil over a high heat. Add the oats, the salt, if desired, and the cinnamon. Stir once, reduce the heat to low, and simmer, uncovered, for 5 minutes without stirring.
2. Add the grated apple and simmer for a further 5 to 7 minutes, stirring only once or twice, until the oatmeal is quite thick. Remove from the heat, cover, and let stand for 10 minutes until very thick.
3. Spoon into warmed bowls, drizzle with the honey, and top each serving with a sprinkling of the raisins.

Oatbran pancakes with warm peach sauce

From the Wyndham Resort and Spa, Florida

Makes 2 servings

½ cup unprocessed oat bran
¼ cup wholewheat flour
2 tsp baking powder
2 tsp sugar
1 tbsp water
¼ cup mashed banana
2 egg whites
½ cup plain non-fat yogurt
orange slices and strawberry fans to garnish

Warm peach sauce
¾ cup unsweetened peach preserve
¾ cup unsweetened apple juice
1 tsp corn starch

1. In a medium bowl, combine the bran, flour, baking powder, and sugar. In a small bowl, stir the water, mashed banana, egg whites, and yogurt until well combined. Pour into the oat bran mixture and stir.
2. Spray a non-stick frying pan or griddle with vegetable oil and place over a medium heat. Pour in ½ cup of the batter for each pancake, allowing room for spreading. Cook until the sides are brown and bubbles form around the edges. Turn and cook until the bottoms are light brown.
3. For the sauce, heat the peach preserve in a small saucepan over a low heat. In a cup, stir the apple juice and corn starch until smooth. Add to the preserve and then bring to the boil, stirring frequently.
4. To serve, place half of the pancakes on each of two plates. Top with the warm peach sauce and garnish with oranges and strawberry fans.

Potato and chive cakes with poached eggs and smoked salmon

from Champneys, Hertfordshire, UK
Makes 4 servings

2½ cups cooked mashed potato
½ cup wholewheat flour
3 tbsp chopped chives
1 tsp crushed coriander seeds
salt and freshly ground black pepper
1 tbsp groundnut or grapeseed oil
1 tbsp white wine vinegar
4 eggs
4 slices of smoked salmon
1 lemon, halved
flat leaf parsley to garnish

1. To make the potato cakes, mix the mashed potato with the flour, chives, and crushed coriander seeds.
2. Season the mixture to taste with salt and pepper and combine to form a firm dough.
3. Roll out on a lightly floured surface to a thickness of ¼-inch. Then, using a 2¾-inch cutter, cut out eight cakes.
4. Heat the oil in a non-stick frying pan and cook the potato cakes until lightly browned—about 3 minutes on each side.
5. Fill a wide, shallow pan halfway with water. Add the vinegar and bring to the boil. Reduce the heat to a gentle simmer and poach the eggs for 3 minutes or until softly poached. Lift out with a slotted spoon and drain on a paper towel.
6. Serve two potato cakes per person with the poached eggs on top and a twist of smoked salmon on the side.
7. Grind black pepper and squeeze a little lemon over the salmon and garnish with parsley.

Blueberry muffins with an apple and cinnamon spread

from Ragdale Hall, Leicestershire, UK
Makes 6 muffins

1 cup wholewheat flour
1 tsp baking powder
1 tbsp low-calorie sweetener
1 large egg, beaten
½ cup skim milk
½ cup fresh blueberries
muffin tin

For the apple and cinnamon spread
2 large cooking apples
1 oz unsalted low-fat margarine
1 tsp clear honey
¼ tsp cinnamon

1. To prepare the muffins, sift the flour, baking powder, and sweetener into a bowl.
2. Make a well in the center and add the beaten egg and milk. Mix well, then carefully stir the blueberries into the muffin mixture, taking care not to break them.
3. Divide the mixture into the muffin tins. Place in a preheated oven at 400°F and bake for 25 to 30 minutes.
4. While the muffins are baking, peel, core, and chop the apples and cook in a saucepan with a little water until soft. Drain off any excess water.
5. Melt the low-fat margarine until runny and stir in the honey. Remove from the heat. Add the apples and cinnamon and blend with a hand-held mixer for 20 seconds until smooth.
6. Place the mixture into the refrigerator to chill and set.
7. Serve the muffins warmed, accompanied by the spread.

Lunch

Most spas share a common philosophy when it comes to food and that is that little and often is the best way of eating. The lunch and dinner recipes are, therefore, interchangeable. You may want to mix and match the soups and salads, have a lighter meal in the evening and a more satisfying lunch, or vice versa–whatever suits your lifestyle, appetite, and time constraints. Just bear in mind that variety is key and use the guidelines at the beginning of the chapter to ensure that you're getting sufficient quantities of the essential nutrients that your body requires.

Gazpacho soup
from Canyon Ranch, Arizona
Makes 8 servings

1 large or 2 small tomatoes
¾ cup peeled diced cucumbers
1 cup mixed diced red and green pepper
¾ cup diced onions
3½ cups low-sodium V8 juice
½ tsp garlic powder
¼ tsp Worcestershire sauce
¼ tsp freshly ground black pepper
2 tbsp freshly squeezed lemon juice
chopped chives, to garnish
2 lemons, cut into 4 wedges

1. Bring a large pot of water to boil. Cut a shallow cross in the top of the tomatoes with a sharp knife. Drop the tomatoes into boiling water for 2 minutes, then transfer to a bowl of iced water. Peel and dice. You should have 1 cup of tomatoes.
2. In a large bowl, combine all the ingredients except the chives and lemons. Mix thoroughly and chill overnight.
3. Serve in chilled bowls and garnish with the chopped chives and lemon wedges.

Watercress, endive, and herb salad with garlic croutons and parmesan in a cider dressing
from Henlow Grange Health Farm, Bedfordshire, UK
Makes 4 servings

For the dressing
1 egg
1 egg yolk
1 tbsp Dijon mustard
1 tbsp cider vinegar
2 cups vegetable oil
8 tbsp dry cider
salt and freshly ground black pepper
1 small baguette
garlic oil

For the salad
2 bunches watercress
7 oz curly endive
2 tbsp chopped, mixed herbs (parsley, chervil, chives, basil, and tarragon)
1 oz Parmesan cheese, grated

1. Whisk the eggs with the mustard and vinegar, and add the vegetable oil. As the dressing becomes thick, thin with the cider. Season with salt and freshly ground black pepper.
2. To make the croutons, slice the baguette very thinly and lightly drizzle with garlic oil. Place into a hot oven and bake at 350°F until golden brown. Remove from the oven, season with salt and pepper, and leave to cool.
3. Put the watercress and endive in a salad bowl and add the herbs, grated Parmesan cheese, and garlic croutons. Coat with the dressing and serve.

Chicken and sugar snap pea stir-fry

from Echo Valley Ranch Resort, Jesmond, Canada
Makes 4 servings

2 tsp corn starch
1 tbsp low-salt soy sauce
3/4 cup chicken stock
2 tsp peanut oil
1 medium onion, chopped
1 medium red pepper, sliced
1/2 cup sugar snap peas
1 lb skinless chicken breast fillets, thinly sliced

1. Dissolve the corn starch in the soy sauce and add to the stock. Set aside. Heat half the oil in a wok, add the onion and pepper, and stir-fry over a high heat until the onion is just soft.
2. Add the peas, stir-fry for a further minute, then remove the vegetables from the wok. Heat the remaining oil in the wok and stir-fry the chicken in batches until browned.
3. Return the vegetables to the wok and add the corn starch, stock, and soy sauce until the mixture boils and thickens.

Carrot and raisin salad

from Canyon Ranch, Arizona, USA
Makes 8 servings

1/2 cup canned crushed pineapple with juice
6 tablespoons non-fat yogurt
6 tablespoons fat-free mayonnaise
2 1/4 lb carrots, grated
1/2 cup raisins

1. Drain the pineapple, reserving the juice. Combine 3 tablespoons of the juice with the yogurt and mayonnaise.
2. Add the pineapple and the carrots and raisins and mix well. Cover tightly and refrigerate, serve cold.

Warm spinach dip with pita chips

from the Professional Golfers Association of America Resort and Spa, Florida
Makes 8 servings

1/4 cup diced onion
1/4 cup diced artichoke hearts
2 tbsp chicken stock
4 oz light cream cheese
1/2 cup non-fat sour cream
2 tbsp rice wine vinegar
ground black pepper
dash of Tabasco sauce
dash of Worcesershire sauce
2 oz chopped fresh spinach
1 oz diced scallions
8 wholewheat pita breads, cut into quarters and toasted

1. In a large saucepan over medium heat, sauté the onion and artichoke hearts in the chicken stock until the onions are translucent.
2. Add the cream cheese and the next five ingredients.
3. Bring to a simmer, stirring constantly.
4. Remove from the heat and stir in the spinach and scallions.
5. Serve warm with toasted pita quarters.

Roasted red potato salad

from Rancho La Puerta, Baja California, Mexico
Makes 6 servings

2 tbsp balsamic vinegar
2 tbsp rice vinegar
2 garlic cloves, minced
1/2 tsp chopped fresh rosemary
pinch hot red pepper flakes (optional)
pinch freshly ground black pepper
1/2 tsp olive oil
4 large red potatoes, cut into 1/2-in pieces
3 hard-boiled large egg whites, chopped
1/2 red onion, diced
1 celery stick, diced
1 medium tomato, diced
1 tsp minced fresh oregano
2 tbsp coarse-grain Dijon mustard
2 tbsp non-fat plain yogurt

1. Preheat the oven to 400°F. Lightly coat a baking sheet or pan with vegetable oil.
2. In a large bowl, combine the vinegars, garlic, rosemary, pepper flakes, pepper, and oil and whisk to mix. Add the potatoes, toss, and then drain the excess marinade, saving 2 tablespoons. Spread the potatoes on the baking sheet and bake for about 45 minutes, until golden brown. It may be necessary to turn the potatoes as they bake to prevent them from burning.
3. In the bowl used to toss the potatoes, combine the egg whites, onion, celery, tomato, oregano, mustard, reserved marinade, and yogurt. Toss the browned, hot potatoes with the ingredients in the bowl. Serve warm or refrigerate for at least 30 minutes to allow the flavors to come together.

Chinese noodle salad

from the Mountain Trek Fitness Retreat and Health Spa, British Columbia, Canada
Makes 4 servings

For the marinade
1/3 cup dark sesame oil
3 tbsp balsamic vinegar
1 tbsp red pepper oil
3 tbsp chopped coriander
1/3 cup soy sauce
3 tbsp sugar
8-10 scallions, thinly sliced
4 cloves garlic, minced
1 tbsp freshly ground ginger

1 x 14 oz package dried Chinese egg or rice noodles

1. Make the marinade by combining the ingredients in a bowl and stirring until the sugar has dissolved.
2. Bring a large pot of water to boil and add the noodles. Stir to prevent sticking. Cook briefly until al dente, then immediately pour the noodles into a colander and rinse with cold water.
3. Shake the colander vigorously to get rid of as much water as possible and put the noodles in a bowl.
4. Stir the marinade again, then pour half of it over the noodles and toss with your hands to distribute evenly. If the noodles aren't to be used immediately, cover with plastic wrap and refrigerate. The flavors and the heat in the red pepper will develop as the noodles stand and the noodles will keep for several days in the refrigerator.
5. Garnish with any raw vegetables, either finely sliced or chopped, such as red pepper, bean sprouts, or snow peas. Add tofu if desired.

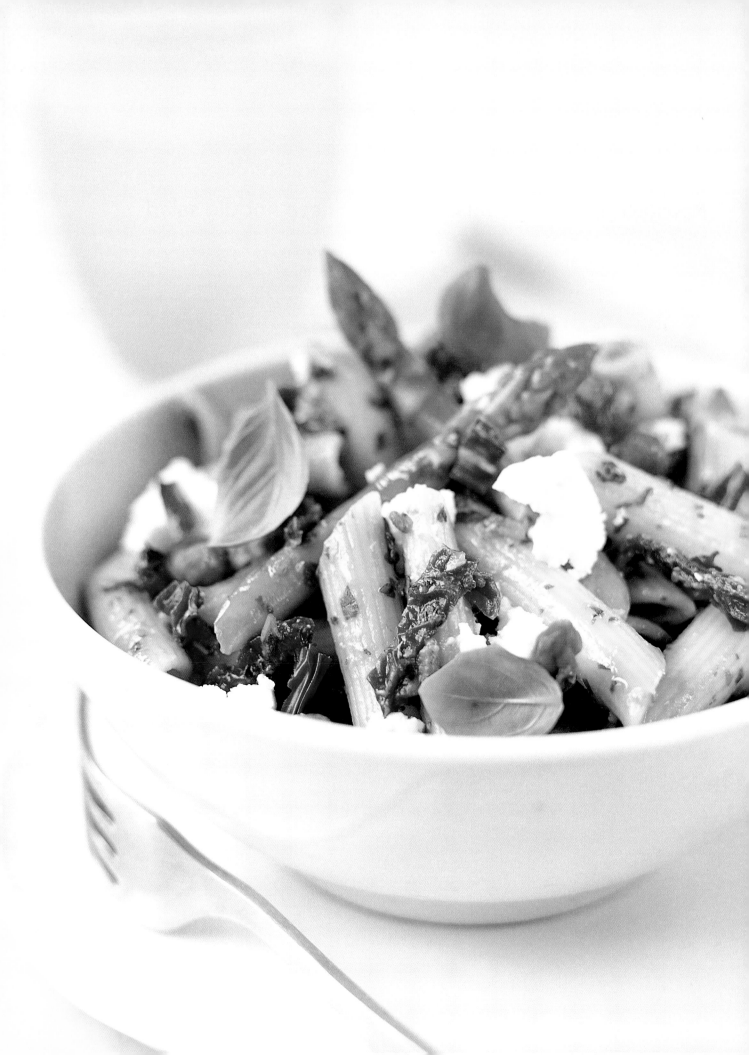

Pasta with sun-dried tomatoes and asparagus in roasted garlic-basil sauce

from Lake Austin Spa Resort, Texas
Makes 4 servings

For the garlic-basil sauce
2 tbsp olive oil
2 heads roasted garlic
7 oz fresh basil, packed
handful of parsley
2 tbsp Parmesan cheese
2 tbsp wine vinegar
freshly ground black pepper
pinch sugar
pinch salt
2 tbsp water

1 cup sun-dried tomatoes, rehydrated, sliced
2 cups blanched asparagus, cut into thirds
julienned zest of one lemon, blanched
5 cups cooked pasta
2 oz feta cheese, crumbled
red pepper flakes

1. First make the garlic-basil sauce. Drizzle a drop or two of olive oil over the garlic, wrap in foil, and roast in the oven at 400°F for 30 minutes.
2. Cool, cut the tops from the heads, and squeeze out. Mix the garlic, basil, and parsley in a food processor.
3. Add the remaining ingredients and process to a thin paste.
4. Rehydrate the sun-dried tomatoes in hot water for 30 minutes. Combine with the asparagus, lemon zest, and pasta. Fold in the basil sauce and add the feta and red pepper.

Caesar salad

from The Golden Door Health Retreat, Queensland, Australia
Makes 4 servings

For the dressing
1 cup plain yogurt
½ cup raw cashews
3-6 cloves garlic
1-2 tbsp lemon juice
1-2 tbsp wholegrain mustard
1-2 tbsp apple juice concentrate
½ tsp sea salt

For the croutons
2 cloves garlic
1 tbsp rosemary
1 tbsp olive oil
½ cup water
sea salt
4 oz diced bread

1 romaine lettuce

1. Combine all the dressing ingredients in a blender and process until smooth. This makes about 2 cups and will keep for 2 months in the refrigerator.
2. For the croutons, blend all the ingredients, except for the diced bread.
3. Toss the diced bread with this mixture and spread on a baking tray. Bake in a hot oven until golden (approximately 10 to 15 minutes).
4. To assemble the salad, chop or tear plenty of romaine lettuce and toss with the croutons and dressing.

Dinner

For most of us, our evening meal is a ritual usually associated with spending time with family or simply having time to ourselves to unwind and reflect on the day. I've selected a handful of my favorite spa recipes for this section–they may need a little more preparation time than the lunch recipes.

New guacamole

from Canyon Ranch, Arizona
Makes 8 servings

½ cup julienned spinach
⅓ cup frozen peas
1 oz lite silken tofu (optional)
1½ tbsp lemon juice
pinch salt
pinch cumin
pinch cayenne
pinch chili powder
dash Tabasco sauce
6 tbsp mashed avocado
3 tbsp peeled and minced tomato
2 tbsp salsa
3 tbsp minced white onions
1 tbsp chopped cilantro
2 tsp chopped scallions

1. Steam the spinach until wilted. Remove from the heat and squeeze out excess water.
2. Then, briefly steam out any remaining excess water.
3. In a food processor, combine the spinach, peas, tofu (if desired), lemon juice, seasonings, and avocado and process until smooth.
4. Fold in the remaining ingredients and mix well.

Chicken fajitas

from Canyon Ranch, Arizona
Makes 4 servings

For the marinade
2 tbsp low-sodium soy sauce
¼ tsp minced ginger root
¼ tsp minced garlic
2 tbsp olive oil
⅓ cup finely chopped coriander
chili powder
3 tbsp beer (optional)
½ tsp Tabasco sauce
½ orange, thinly sliced
½ lemon, thinly sliced
½ lime, thinly sliced
1 tbsp parsley

4 boneless, skinless chicken breast halves
1 cup sliced assorted capsicum
4 flour tortillas (9 in diameter)
½ cup new guacamole (see left)
½ cup salsa
½ cup fat-free sour cream

1. Combine the marinade ingredients in a shallow baking dish and mix well.
2. Cover the chicken breasts with the marinade, turning to coat evenly. Cover and refrigerate for at least 2 hours or overnight.
3. Lift the breasts from the marinade and grill for 3 to 5 minutes per side.
4. While the chicken is grilling, lightly spray a medium frying pan with non-stick vegetable oil. Over a medium heat, sauté the pepper strips until just tender. Keep warm.
5. Cut each chicken breast into strips and serve with a tortilla, some of the peppers, and 2 tablespoons each of guacamole, salsa, and fat-free sour cream.

Ancho chile-dusted eggplant parmesan with slow-roasted garden tomatoes

from Westward Look Resort, Arizona
Makes 6 servings

6 large vine-ripe tomatoes
1 oz chopped cilantro
1 oz chopped parsley
3 medium eggplants
salt
freshly ground black pepper
2 cups sourdough breadcrumbs
4 oz grated parmesan cheese
1 tbsp ancho chile powder
2 eggs
½ cup milk
1 cup all-purpose flour
2 tbsp olive oil

1. Wash and core the tomatoes, then cut them in half. Place them cut side up on a baking sheet. Season with salt and freshly ground black pepper. Rub with a thin layer of olive oil and sprinkle with a quarter of the chopped herbs.
2. Place the tomatoes in the oven and slow roast at 250°F for approximately 1 hour.
3. Just before the tomatoes are ready, slice the eggplant into disks, season with salt and freshly ground black pepper, and set aside. In a small mixing bowl, combine the breadcrumbs, parmesan cheese, the rest of the chopped herbs, and ancho chili powder.
4. In another shallow bowl, scramble the eggs with the milk and set aside. To coat the eggplant, lightly dust with flour, dip in the egg wash, and then coat with the breading. In a large pan set over medium heat, sauté the eggplant in the olive oil for about 3 minutes on both sides until golden brown.

Fresh fish steaks with herbs, lemon, garlic, mushrooms, and cocktail potatoes

from the Hyatt Regency-Coolum, Queensland, Australia
Makes 4 servings

9 oz roasting potatoes, peeled
7 oz wild mushrooms
juice of 4 medium lemons
1 tsp peeled, crushed garlic
1 tsp parsley
4 tomatoes
4 fresh salmon or tuna steaks
1 tbsp olive oil
1½ cups boiled brown rice
1½ cups baby carrots, peeled and cooked
1 lemon, cut into 4 wedges
handful watercress, to garnish

1. Roast the potatoes.
2. Steam the mushrooms whole for 6 minutes, remove from steamer, and keep the remaining liquid.
3. Slice the mushrooms thinly and add to the mushroom liquid along with the lemon juice, crushed garlic and chopped parsley.
4. Cut the tomatoes in quarters, remove the seeds, and cut into small pieces. Then add to the mushrooms. Set aside.
5. Clean the fish and pan-fry in olive oil on both sides.
6. Cut the roasted potatoes in half and place in the frying pan with the fish. Finish in the oven at 350°F until cooked (around 8 minutes depending on the fish used).
7. Place the potatoes, boiled rice, and cooked baby carrots on the bottom of the plate. Put the fish on top of the potatoes. Finish by spooning the mushroom and tomato mixture over the top, and garnish with lemon and sprigs of watercress.

Purple basil risotto with parmesan shavings

from The Spa at Rajvilas, Jaipur, India
Makes 4 servings

½ cup red peppers
½ cup yellow peppers
2 oz parmesan cheese
2 tbsp olive oil
1 cup shallots, chopped
2 tsp chopped garlic
2 cups Arborio rice
2½ cups water
½ cup white wine
2½ oz butter
salt
freshly ground black pepper
1 oz purple basil

1. Grill and dice the peppers.
2. Grate the parmesan cheese and put evenly on a medium hot pan, cool, and remove.
3. Heat the oil and sweat the shallots and garlic. Add the Arborio rice and cook with water till just done (as described on the packet).
4. Add the white wine and butter and check seasoning.
5. Purée three-quarters of the basil and add to the rice together with the diced pepper.
6. Garnish with the remaining basil, chopped, and parmesan shavings.

Roasted fillets of cod with mango and tomato salsa

from Champneys, Hertfordshire, UK
Makes 4 servings

For the mango and tomato salsa
½ mango, peeled and finely diced
1 small red onion, finely diced
2 ripe red tomatoes, peeled, seeded, and diced
2 ripe yellow tomatoes, peeled, seeded, and diced
1 garlic clove, finely chopped
1 bunch chives, chopped
1 tbsp sugar
2 tsp extra virgin olive oil
1 tbsp sherry vinegar
dash sweet chili sauce

2 bunches asparagus
2 tbsp olive oil
4 young cod fillets (about 5 oz each) with skin, scaled, and boned
2 lb baby spinach or Swiss chard
salt and freshly ground pepper

1. First make the salsa. Place the mango, onion, and tomatoes in a bowl. Add the remaining ingredients, mix, and refrigerate.
2. Heat the oven to 400°F and put a baking sheet in the oven to heat up.
3. Trim the asparagus into 2-inch pieces and, if necessary, trim the thick part of the stem with a peeler. Steam for 5 minutes.
4. Heat the olive oil in a non-stick frying pan. Add the fish fillets, flesh side down, and fry for 2 minutes. Place the fish skin side down on the preheated baking sheet, add the asparagus, and roast in the hot oven for 7 minutes.
5. Using the same frying pan, stir-fry the spinach or chard until tender. Drain and season to taste. Place the spinach in the center of four serving plates, pile the asparagus on top and lastly the crisp-skinned fish. Serve with salsa around the side.

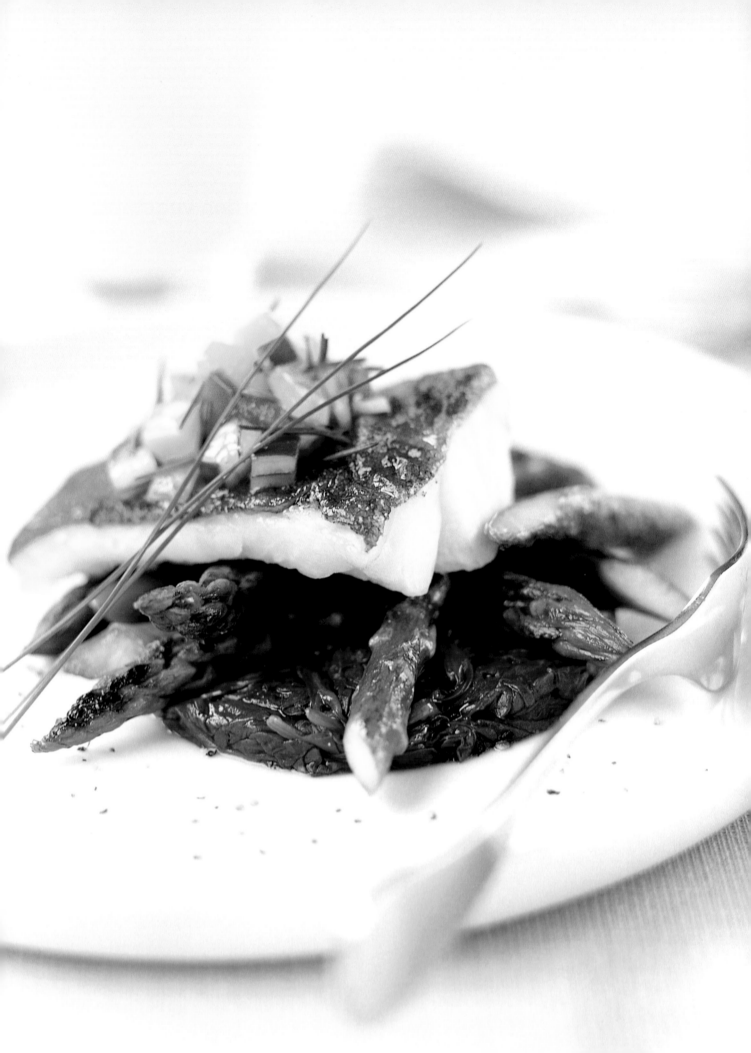

Indonesian chicken with grilled bananas

from Canyon Ranch, Arizona
Makes 4 servings

For the dry rub mix
½ tsp ground ginger
1 tsp ground cayenne pepper
½ tsp ground allspice
½ tsp ground cinnamon
1 tsp ground curry powder
1 tsp ground paprika
½ tsp ground turmeric
¼ tsp salt

4 boneless chicken breast halves, all fat removed
2 bananas
1 tbsp light brown sugar

1. Combine all the dry rub ingredients and mix well. Lightly coat each chicken breast with the rub. Place on a plate and cover tightly. Refrigerate for at least 1 hour before grilling.
2. Pre-heat the grill. Slice the bananas in half lengthwise, skins left on. Sprinkle the brown sugar on the bananas and rub it in as much as possible. Grill the bananas lightly, cut side down. Remove from the heat and set aside.
3. Remove the chicken from the refrigerator and place on the grill. Grill for about 5 minutes on each side until done.
4. Serve each grilled chicken breast with a grilled banana half still in the peel.

Grilled garden vegetable platter

from Westward Look Resort, Arizona
Makes 8 servings

1 bunch Italian parsley
1 tbsp fresh thyme leaves
3 cloves of garlic, freshly chopped
1 tbsp crushed red pepper flakes
freshly ground black pepper to taste
2 cups olive oil
2 medium zucchini
2 medium yellow squash
4 medium tomatoes
2 green chilies
2 red peppers
salt

1. Rinse the parsley, pat dry, and then finely chop.
2. Pick the fresh thyme leaves from the stems. In a bowl, add the parsley and thyme, and mix together with the garlic, red pepper flakes, freshly ground black pepper, and olive oil.
3. Slice the vegetables into ½-inch-thick long slices. Toss the vegetables with enough marinade to coat lightly. Let them chill in the refrigerator for about an hour.
4. Remove the vegetables from the bowl and place flat on a baking sheet pan and season to taste with salt and freshly ground black pepper.
5. Transfer the vegetables to the grill, and grill over a high heat for approximately 1½ minutes on each side, or until desired crispness.
6. Place back on the rinsed baking sheet to chill to room temperature. Serve as appetizers.

Smooth delights

We all like the occasional treat, but all too often it's in the form of a fat- and calorie-packed package of chips or a chocolate bar. There's nothing wrong with having the odd indulgence but if you are trying to re-educate your palette and detox your system, why not try some of the health-conscious treats on offer at the world's leading health spas and resorts.

Banana, citrus, and oat smoothie

from Champneys, Hertfordshire, UK
Makes 4 servings

½ cup rolled oats
⅓ cup skim milk
3 small bananas
finely grated zest and juice of 1 orange
finely grated zest and juice of 1 lemon
1 cup low-fat yogurt
3 tbsp clear honey
pinch mixed spice
8 ice cubes

1. Put the oats in a bowl, add the milk, and leave to soak overnight in the refrigerator.
2. Keep the fruit, yogurt, and fromage frais in the refrigerator overnight.
3. In the morning, chop the bananas and place in a blender with the oats and all the remaining ingredients. Blend until smooth, then pass through a fine sieve and serve in chilled glasses with ice and straws.

Banana smoothie

from Lucknam Park, Wiltshire, UK
Makes 1 serving

7 oz bananas
¾ cup low-fat 2% milk
1 tbsp natural yogurt
2 tbsp clear honey
½ cup vanilla ice cream
4 ice cubes

1. Combine all the ingredients in a food processor or blender and blend until smooth. Serve in a chilled glass.

Paradise punch

from Canyon Ranch, Arizona
Makes 1 serving

½ cup skim milk
½ cup unsweetened pineapple juice
2 tbsp non-fat cottage cheese
½ tsp sugar
¼ tsp vanilla extract
¼ tsp coconut extract
2 ice cubes

1. Combine all the ingredients in a food processor or blender and blend until smooth. Serve in a chilled glass.

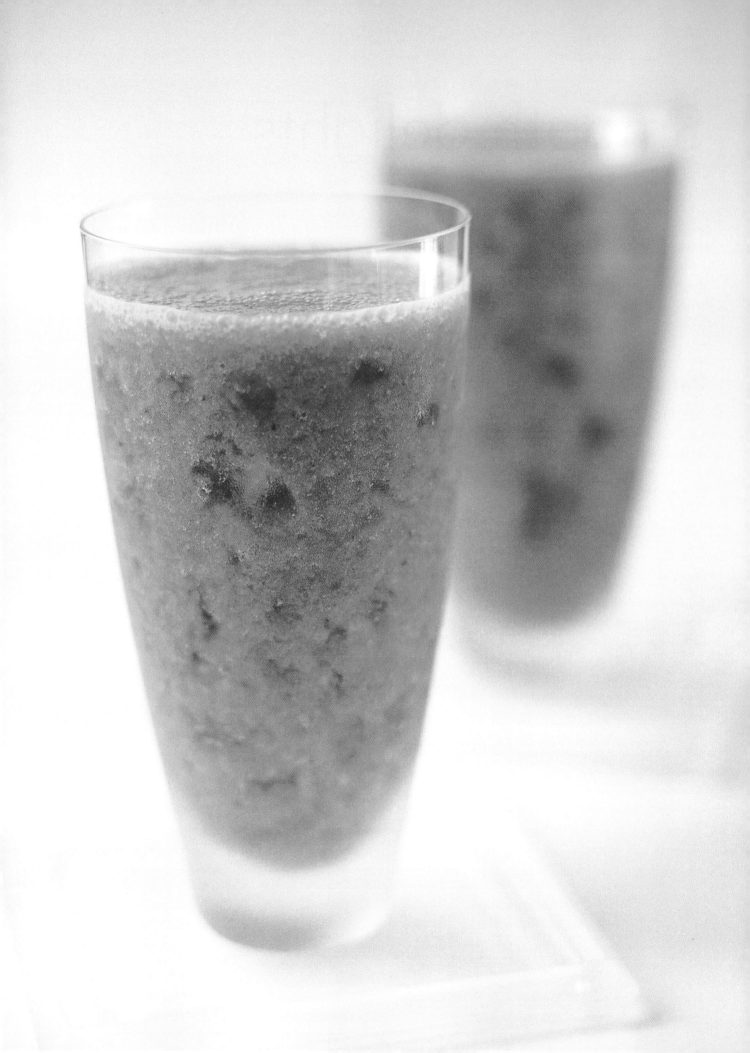

Strawberry-banana smoothie

from Rancho La Puerta, Baja California, Mexico
Makes 2 servings

14 oz hulled strawberries
2 bananas
1 cup unsweetened, unfiltered apple juice
2 to 3 tbsp fresh lime juice
ice cubes
mint leaves to garnish

1. Combine all the ingredients except the mint leaves in a food processor and blend until smooth. Pour into glasses, garnish with mint leaves, and serve immediately.

Energizer smoothie

from the Golden Door, California
Makes 2 servings

¾ cup fresh orange juice
¾ cup low-fat plain yogurt
1 banana
4 to 5 pitted dates, cut into pieces
1 tbsp wheat or oat germ

1. Combine all the ingredients in a food processor and blend until smooth and creamy. Serve immediately.

Original golden door potassium broth

from the Golden Door, California
Makes 12 servings

This is one of my all-time favorite brews, reminding me of my first trip to the Golden Door spa and my morning hike up the mountain. As Michel Stroot, executive chef at the spa, explains, potassium broth is incredibly replenishing if you've been exercising and is an energy boost. "Potassium, available in fruits and vegetables, is an important mineral that needs replenishing after an energetic workout, when it is lost. [As much as 500 to 600 milligrams are lost after two or three hours of strenuous exercise.] This is why we serve this mid-morning by the pool after our guests have hiked, weight-trained, and participated in aerobic classes. They need it! And they love it."

12 to 14 plum tomatoes, quartered, or 1 x 1-lb, 12-oz can crushed plum tomatoes
14 oz chopped vegetable trimmings, such as celery stalks and leaves, onions, carrots, cabbage, peppers, and parsley stems
2 garlic cloves, crushed
1 tbsp dried basil or chopped fresh basil leaves
1 tsp red pepper flakes (optional)

1. In a large saucepan, combine the tomatoes, vegetable trimmings, garlic, basil, pepper flakes (if using), and 3½ pints of water and bring to a boil over a high heat. Reduce the heat and simmer, uncovered, for about 45 minutes until the flavors blend.
2. Strain the broth through a sieve, gently pressing on the solids to extract as much flavor as possible. Discard the solids. Serve hot.

Desserts

The idea that health spas and desserts do not go together is, quite frankly, a myth. Providing that you stick to moderate portions and don't go overboard, a dessert is the ideal way to complete a meal. I've gathered my personal favorites from a host of mouth-watering temptations from the top ranking spas across the globe. Naturally, they are only a taster of what you will find at a spa but they do make you realize that you can have something sweet.

Strawberry cheesecake

from Henlow Grange Health Farm, Bedfordshire, UK
Makes 4 servings

¾ cup muesli
½ cup apple juice
2 tsp all-purpose flour
½ cup strawberry purée
⅓ cup low-fat cream cheese
⅓ cup natural yogurt
2 tsp sweetener
4 tsp gelatin powder
1 lb strawberries

1. Line four ramekins with parchment paper. Mix the muesli, apple juice, and flour and press into the ramekins.
2. Combine the purée, cream cheese, natural yogurt, and sweetener and set with the gelatin.
3. Pour into the ramekins and refrigerate.
4. Serve decorated with fresh strawberries.

Carrot cake

from Canyon Ranch, Arizona
Makes 24 servings

2½ cup wholewheat flour
1½ tsp baking powder
1½ tsp cinnamon
pinch salt
4 egg yolks
5 tbsp sunflower oil
¼ cup buttermilk
¼ cup fructose
1½ tsp vanilla extract
⅔ cup chopped walnuts, toasted
2½ cup grated carrots
1¾ crushed pineapple, drained
6 egg whites
¼ cup fructose
pinch baking powder
1½ tsp corn oil margarine
1½ tsp corn syrup
6 tbsp buttermilk
1½ tsp vanilla extract

1. Preheat the oven to 325°F and coat a 9- x 13-inch pan with a non-stick vegetable spray. Sift the flour, baking powder, cinnamon, and salt into a large bowl.
2. In a medium bowl, combine the egg yolks, oil, buttermilk, fructose, and vanilla. Add to the flour mixture and stir in until combined. Stir in the walnuts, carrots, and pineapple.
3. In a small bowl, beat six egg whites until they hold a peak. Fold into the batter. Pour the mixture into the pan and bake for 30 to 35 minutes. The cake is done when it springs back when pushed in at the center. Remove from the oven and cool.
4. For the glaze, combine the remaining ingredients, except the vanilla, in a saucepan and bring to the boil. Reduce the heat and simmer for 5 minutes. Remove the glaze from the heat and stir in the vanilla. Use a fork to poke holes in the top of the cake. Pour the glaze over the warm cake.

Filo pastry apple strudel

from the Golden Door, California
Makes 6 servings

This is simply the best apple strudel I've ever tasted and even more pleasure was derived from it by learning to make it in the kitchen of the Golden Door itself. Part of the spa's program includes an evening cookery class where you can learn some of the spa's best-loved recipes so that you can take home a little piece for yourself–literally. Even if you're not a big dessert fan, don't miss this one.

5 Golden Delicious apples, peeled, cored, and sliced
2 tsp ground cinnamon
pinch ground cloves
¼ cup raisins or dried cranberries
½ cup brown sugar
five 12- x 17-in sheets of filo pastry
confectioners' sugar for sprinkling

1. Coat a large non-stick sauté pan with vegetable oil spray and sauté the apples with the cinnamon, cloves, raisins, and brown sugar over a medium heat for 8 to 10 minutes, stirring frequently, until the apples begin to soften. Transfer to a bowl to cool.
2. Preheat the oven to 350°F and coat a baking sheet with vegetable oil spray.
3. Place one sheet of the filo pastry on a work surface with a long side towards you and spray it with vegetable oil spray. Stack the remaining filo sheets on top, spraying each sheet. Spoon the apple filling in a long row across the center of the dough. Starting with the long side facing you, roll up the dough around the filling to enclose it. Tuck in the ends and transfer to the baking sheet, seam side down.
4. Lightly spray the top of the roll with vegetable oil spray. Bake for 35 to 40 minutes, until the pastry is golden brown. Sprinkle with confectioners' sugar, cut into slices, and serve warm.

Berry compote

from The Greenhouse, Texas
Makes 12 servings

8 oz fresh raspberries
6 oz fresh blueberries
8 oz fresh strawberries cut into quarters
2 tbsp orange zest
4 oz raspberries, fresh or frozen
2 tbsp sugar-free strawberry fruit jam
½ banana, peeled

1. Place the fresh raspberries, blueberries, strawberries, and orange zest into a bowl.
2. Place the additional fresh or frozen raspberries, the fruit jam, and banana into a food processor and blend until smooth. Strain the mixture if desired.
3. Add the puréed mixture to the berries and orange zest mixture and toss gently. Keep refrigerated.

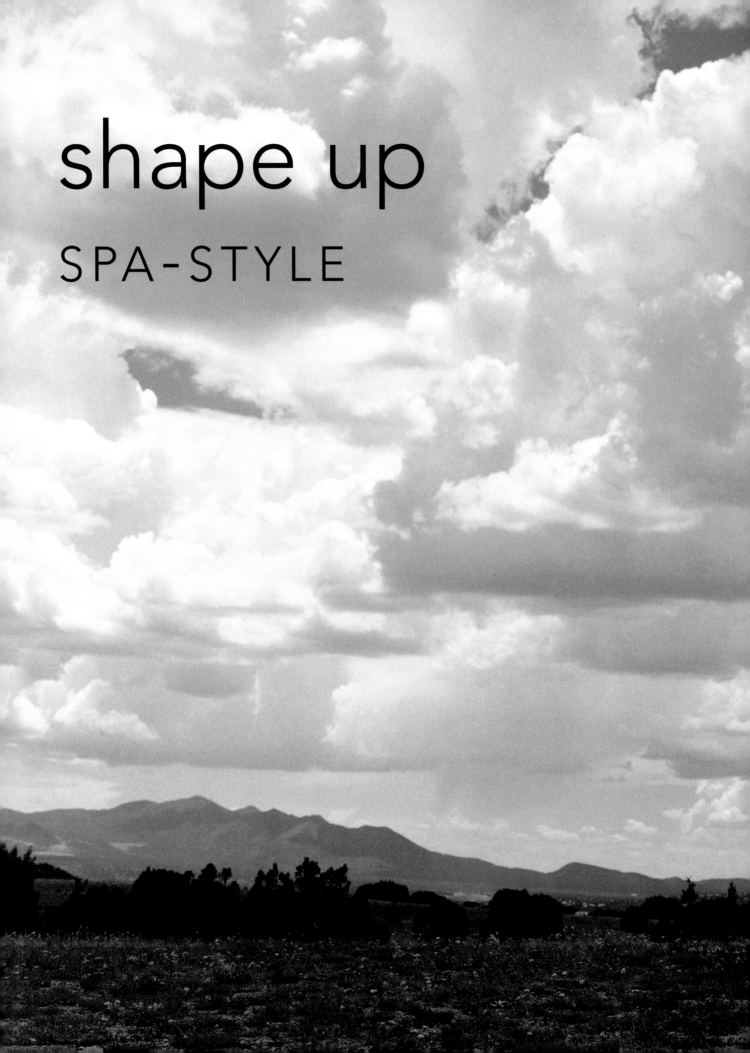

shape up
SPA-STYLE

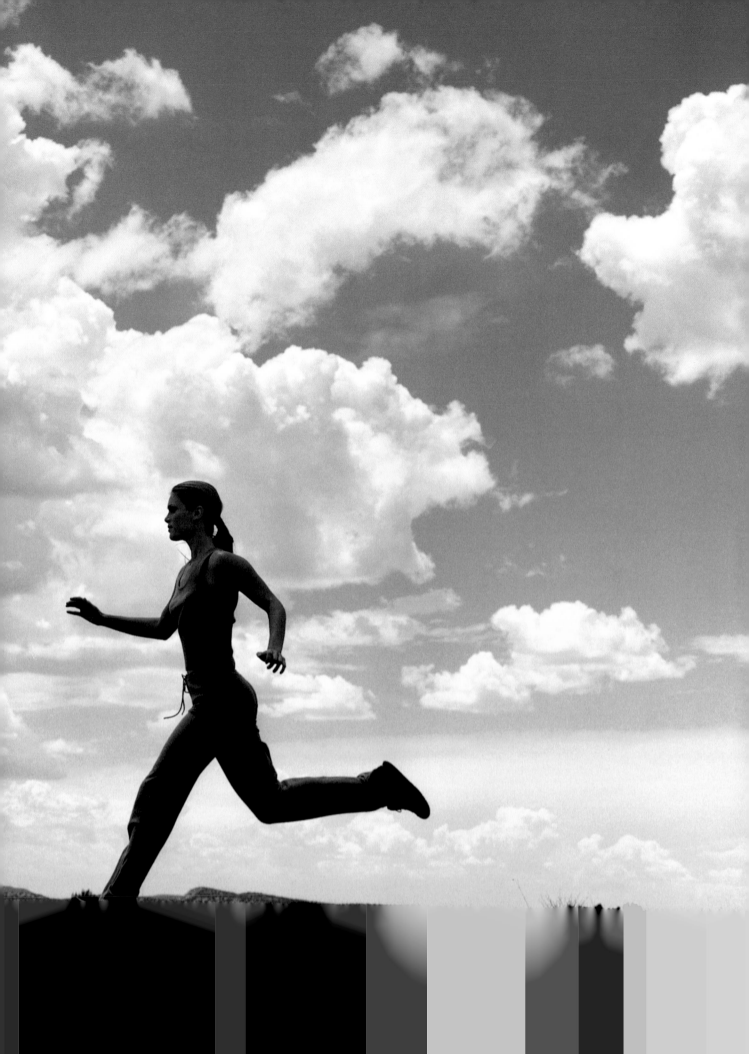

Time to get going

Part of the pleasure of checking into a spa is the knowledge that, with a little bit of effort, you can check out a week later not only looking better but feeling healthier and actually being fitter. A spa break is often the vital kick-start that we need to motivate us from a passive state to an active one. Let's be honest. It's all too easy to become a couch potato at home when you expend so much of your energy at work, and leisure time just doesn't seem to have a place in your busy never-rest-for-a-minute lifestyle. While a spa break may not fit into your schedule at this moment, you can benefit from the fitness expertise available at the world's top spas.

Going to the gym is often the last thing any of us wants to do at the end of a frenetic day and even though we know it does us good, we just don't seem to have the motivation. The solution? We've asked the experts from the international spas—the Golden Door, California; Echo Valley Ranch, Jesmond, Canada; and St. David's Hotel, Cardiff; Henlow Grange Health Farm, Bedfordshire; and Ragdale Hall Health Hydro, Leicestershire, UK—to share their fitness secrets, motivation tricks, and get-you-back-in-shape moves so you can get on track. From walking to weight training, spa fitness experts give their advice on activities that you can do easily at home. And to increase your flexibility, there are stretching exercises to tone your muscles.

From boosting your immune system to relieving stress and reducing depression, there are a million good reasons to exercise. A recent government report suggested that even thirty minutes of physical activity each day would lead to significant improvements in health and well being. These include a reduction in the risk of strokes and developing heart disease, non-insulin dependent diabetes, and hip fractures due to osteoporosis. Exercise also helps to improve brain function, lower blood cholesterol and blood pressure levels, and it promotes sounder sleep.

CREATE YOUR OWN EXERCISE PROGRAM

An effective exercise program, according to the experts at The Spa at St. David's Hotel, needs to promote aerobic endurance, flexibility, and strength. Thankfully, aerobic endurance exercise doesn't mean that you need to run a marathon. You can change aspects of your lifestyle to fit aerobic endurance into your life as well as setting aside time for training. For example, instead of taking the bus or train to work, cycle or walk or, if walking the whole way isn't an option, get off the bus or train a few stops early and walk the rest of the way. Even small sacrifices, like walking up and down the stairs instead of taking the elevator every day, will help.

One of the biggest hurdles to get over is actually motivating yourself to begin and then stick to an exercise program. So, here, Dean L. Hodgkin, a global Reebok trainer and consultant to Ragdale Hall Health Hydro, shares his motivational tips, guaranteed to get you off the couch, once and for all:

1. FOCUS

It is time to move but so often thinking about doing it is what is difficult. It is always easier once you get going. (Ever had a day when the journey to the gym was harder than the workout?) So make a start as soon as possible.

Commit yourself to improving with every fiber of your being and you will be amazed at how many hurdles you can overcome. If you are not really committed, you might as well give up, as you are unlikely to see great results.

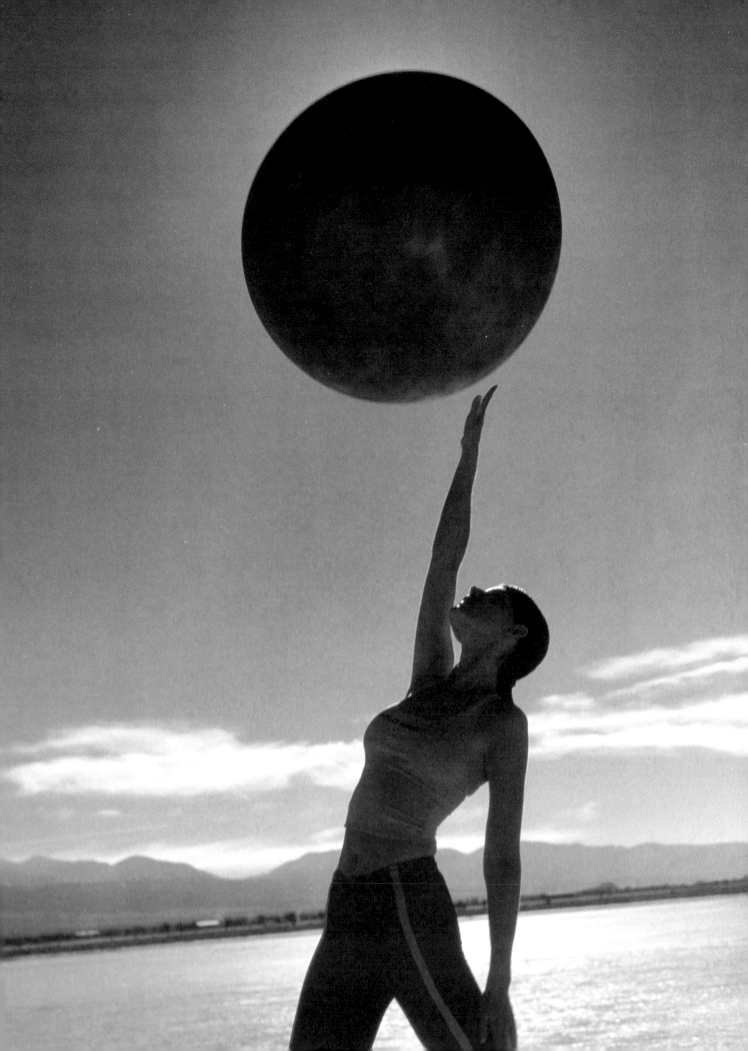

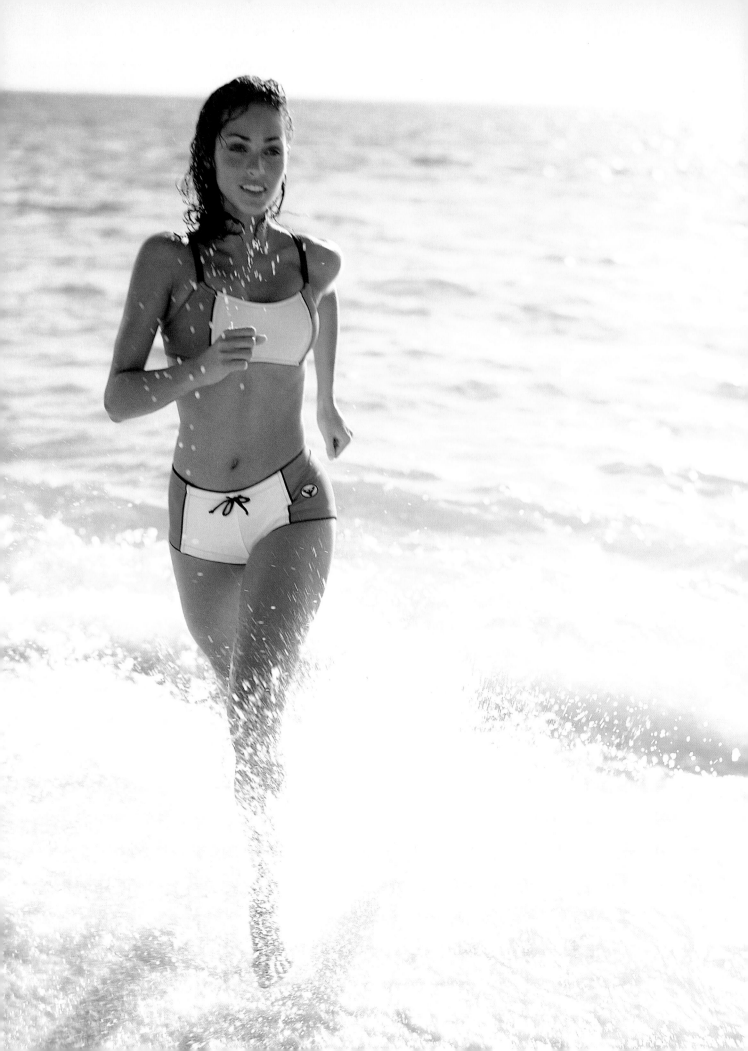

2. THINK POSITIVELY

From the outside, life will always present obstacles, which have to be worked around, under, over, or through if you are truly committed to getting fitter. But it is all too easy to sabotage progress from the inside with that small voice that says, "You'll never make it," or the perverse part of our nature that holds us back from doing whatever it takes to move on. Look to beat this self-defeating behavior by replacing it with more constructive thought patterns. Think positive and you are far more likely to achieve what you set out to do.

If you feel overwhelmed by the enormity of your task, remember that before you know it small steps will add up to big steps. Take one step at a time and congratulate yourself after every one. Your prize awaits you. To help set yourself some goals see right, and then check regularly that what you are doing is taking you closer to reaching them. If it is not, you need to adapt your goals, which of course is fine. Try to do something each day that helps you to reach your goals.

Zap any negative thoughts with the power of positive thinking. Tell yourself daily that you will achieve your goal, and visualize yourself winning through any adversity and enjoying the rewards reaching your goals will bring you.

Spend time with positive people too (not everyone will agree that your goals are possible or be happy that you are changing). Friends that support you and colleagues that motivate you will prove invaluable in your desire to change. Sharing your workouts with someone can be fun and you can inspire each other to keep going.

If you know someone who has already achieved what you are setting out to do, decide if what worked for them will work for you. By adopting their habits you may save yourself time –they will have taken some of the trial and error out for you!

It may also help you to move forward if you remember how you achieved other difficult things in the past, but that you did what it took and you got there in the end.

3. LIVE AND LEARN

There will be times when things do not go according to plan and you do not move on as much as you would like. If you have lost your focus, review your goals. Thinking about how much you will enjoy achieving them will put you back in the game again. If it's a mistake that is getting you down, try thinking of it simply as a result you created through a certain action. If you change the action you will create a new result.

SETTING GOALS

If you are not exactly sure what you want, spend some time asking yourself these questions:
• What would you do if you knew you couldn't fail?
• What do you love doing?
• What skills do you already have that help you to be successful?
• What will the year ahead be like if you don't take the next step?
• Once you have decided on your goal, or goals, write them down (yes, committing them to paper really does help!). Then set yourself a realistic time frame for each goal and decide how to start moving towards them.
• Be specific–if you are not sure where you are going, you may not like where you end up! Exactly what do you want to achieve? What will this feel like? What difference will this make in your life?

Mix and match

No two bodies are the same so the chances are that an exercise program that is right for someone else may not work for you. The secret to sticking to an exercise regime is to find one that's personalized to you. It goes without saying that a trip to a spa or going to the gym regularly will give you a head start. A qualified fitness instructor can help you work out a schedule that suits your lifestyle. But the good news is that you can get on to the right track yourself by following a few golden rules. Fitness expert Julie Pelletier, from Echo Valley Ranch Resort in Jesmond, Canada, shares her tips and training know-how.

Pelletier says that one of the most common mistakes we make when we begin an exercise program is to exercise too much. At the beginning, we tend to be very motivated and exercise four or more times a week when for years that's as much as we were doing in a whole year. So in terms of long-term motivation, start very slowly, maybe working out twice a week, and not more, even if you want to. If you can maintain this over a one-month period, then add one workout per week. It is far better to exercise twice a week for an extended period than to exercise six times a week for three weeks and then stop because of lack of motivation or injury. People can't expect to go from zero workouts per week to playing tennis or jogging four times a week without suffering injuries. The body has to be able to adapt. And it doesn't happen overnight.

Another common situation that causes a decrease in interest is that people often do the same workout over and over again. That's where a technique called Cross Training

KICK-START YOURSELF

Here's an example of a kick-start fitness program to take you from couch potato to regular exerciser. Begin by committing to working out twice a week.
• 15 minutes of aerobic exercise such as walking or cycling.
• 10 minutes strengthening stretches.
Then you should feel able to take on more strenuous forms of exercise on a regular basis. Just take that initial step and you will soon find yourself getting into the swing of things.

comes into play, which involves doing a variety of physical activities. On Monday, go to a park for a walk. On Wednesday, do home weight training. On Thursday, go biking. And on Saturday, try a jog-walk mix (see Cross Training ideas overleaf). In this way, you avoid doing the same thing all the time. By being active in various ways, the risk of getting injured diminishes and multiple muscles are being used. And in this way, if it's raining on Monday, you can switch to an indoor weight training session. Or if you don't feel like biking on Wednesday, you can take a walk instead. Do what you feel like doing.

Instead of going to the gym on Saturday morning, why not go ice-skating on Saturday night or find a local boat club and try kayaking. If it's too hot and humid to go for a jog, go to a local pool and do your jogging program in the pool, in either deep or shallow water.

ACTIVITY GUIDE

Want to find the activity best suited to your fitness requirements? Fitness expert, Dean L. Hodgkin, gives the lowdown on the top spa fitness activities that are also suitable for at-home or health club practice. We have then taken the first three suggestions–stretching, weight training and walking–and provided you with programs on pages 78–83 to get you underway.

Strengthening stretches (see pages 78–9): Doing strengthening stretches for 10 minutes twice a week is not much, but it is much better than nothing. You could also include some exercises during a walk: when you pass some steps, do some heel raises; when you pass a tree, do push-ups against it, and when you pass a bench, do step-ups. Finish with abdominal exercises and more stretching at home.

Weight training (see pages 80–1): This is the best form of exercise to change your body shape and it will speed up your metabolic rate, meaning your body will burn up more calories, even while you sleep. It is important to get a trainer to teach you safe techniques and to ensure the program is balanced, to reduce any risk of injury. A huge plus is that bones strengthen, reducing the risk of osteoporosis.

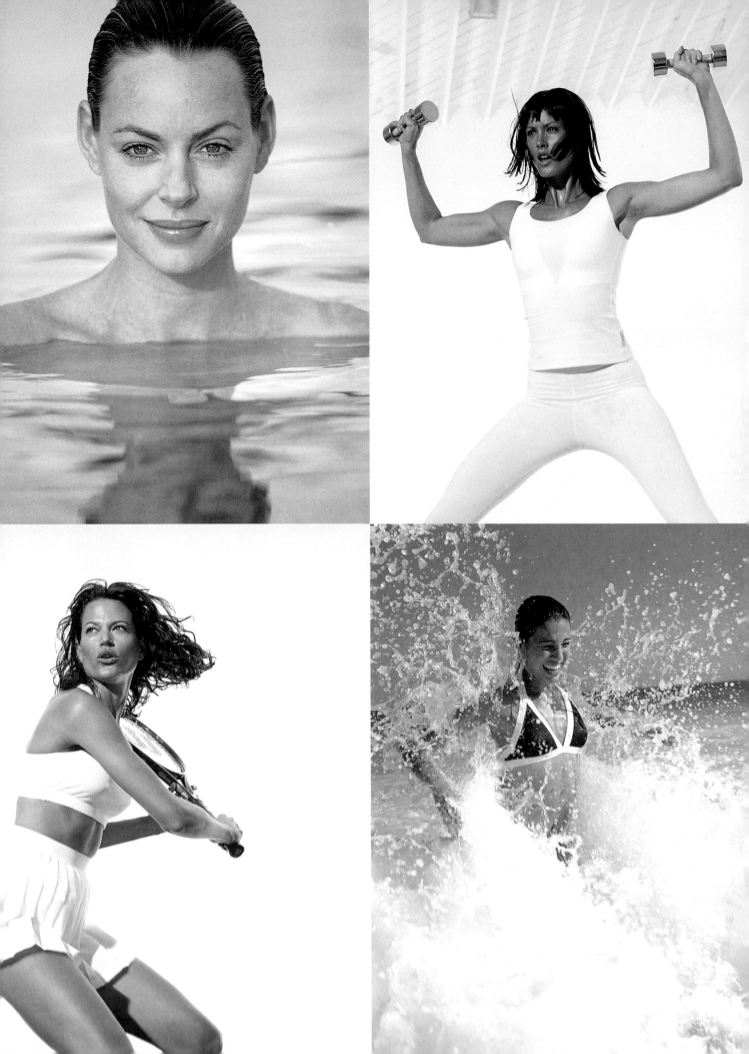

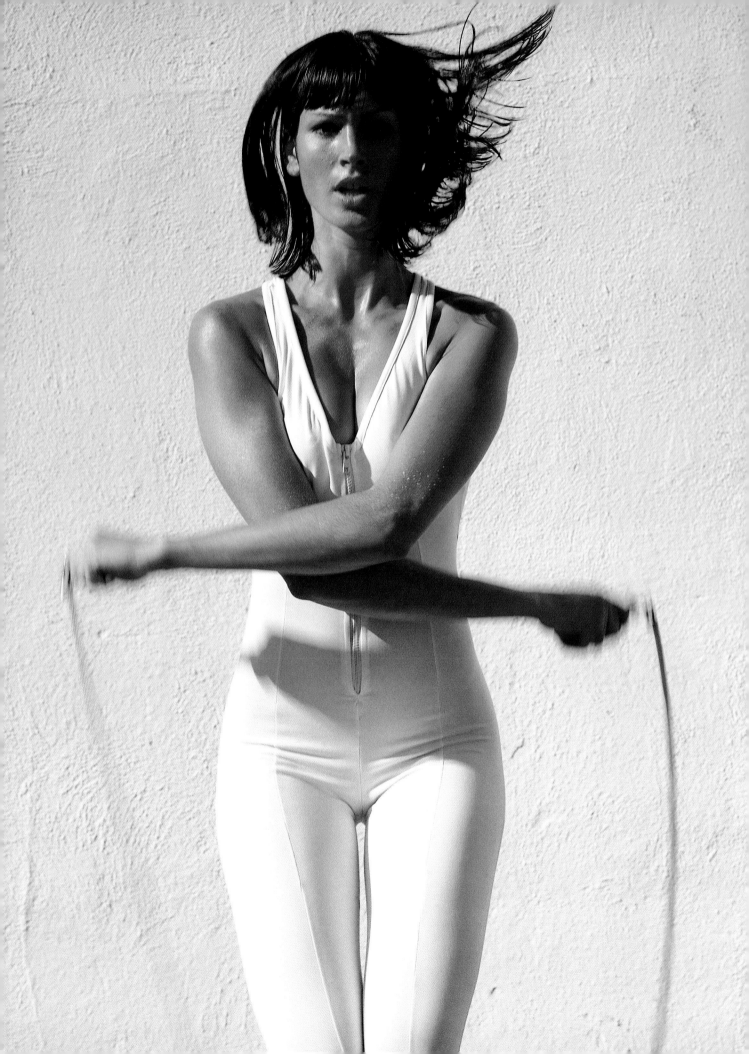

Power walking (see pages 82–3): This exercise is a fantastic way of getting fit because it is so accessible, whatever your age or fitness level. A great component in weight-loss programs, power walking has been shown to have considerable stress-reducing properties related to the endorphin "high," which is more pronounced when exercise is done outdoors. It is a great choice for anyone who is overweight as the stress in the joints is reduced but you can still achieve a suitable intensity level by varying the pace in intervals or introducing inclines.

Swimming: This is a triple whammy because it is a good calorie consumer, improves the efficiency of the heart and lungs, and helps to tone the whole body due to the resistive properties of the exercise medium–water. The best thing about this activity is that due to the cooling and comforting effects of the water, you tend not to feel as if you are working as hard as in the gym or a class. To get the most out of it, forget the breaststroke and go for the crawl.

Canoeing: It helps prevent lower back trouble by forcing you to use your core (trunk) strength muscles, due to sitting upright with legs out in front. The shoulders, arms, and upper back will get magnificent toning. It's harder in the sea than in still water but either way a good sense of balance is a prerequisite.

Biking: While stationary bikes are now very popular, opt for getting out, as there are noticeable mood improvements from changing scenery and interacting with nature. It has good potential for burning calories but toning is limited to the lower body. Overdoing it may lead to kyphotic (round shoulder) characteristics, so try to balance biking with a good post-exercise stretch.

Tennis: It is not too useful in weight loss as there is a lot of stopping and starting, but it can be a great way to vent aggression in a harmless way. Tennis has super toning effects for the legs but over time can take its toll on the hips, knees, and ankles. Since it is a unilateral activity, other sessions will be required to balance stresses in the musculoskeletal system.

CROSS TRAINING

To vary your workout, try some of the following ideas:

Jog/walk mix or walk/skip mix: Jogging improves aerobic fitness but as it is high impact, it can place stress on the joints. So ensure that you have a very good pair of shoes with ample shock absorption. Jogging provides great toning for the lower body and is an excellent calorie burner but use it in tandem with other exercises to achieve all-round improvements. Here's how:

Do a mix of jogging and walking. For a beginner, walk 5 minutes as a warm-up. Then jog 2 minutes and walk 3 minutes and repeat 4 times, then 10 minutes normal walking. Any other pattern is also fine. If you want to increase the jogging portion, you can move to 2 minutes of jogging and 2 minutes of walking. Work up to a full 20 minutes of jogging. Think safely–do not run alone at night in areas that are not well lit.

Give it some rope: Skipping is a very good cardiovascular exercise, but in reality, who wants to be skipping for 20 minutes–or who can? One way to integrate skipping into a workout could be to go for a 30 minutes walk and incorporate four periods of skipping into it. It would increase the intensity of the walk and probably make it more challenging. Try skipping for 1 minute without mistakes, try beating your own record, or skipping without mistake longer than your friend.

Take the stairs: Another way to increase the intensity of a walk and work on your thighs and buttock muscles would be to do "stairs"–if your park or gym has some. Go up and down the stairs a few times. If you are agile enough, take two stairs at a time. Very good for strengthening the legs.

Stretch and strengthen

Stretching is a very important aspect of a fitness program. When given proper stretching exercises, people with lower back, neck, elbow, or knee problems can find the pain diminishes. One study found that eighty percent of people will have back pain at some point during their lives. So as a preventive tool or as part of a treatment, stretching can be used. The best way to learn proper technique is to consult an exercise specialist, such as an athletic therapist or sports physiotherapist. Then you can do it on your own. A lot of exercises can be done at work while sitting in front of a computer or while watching television. Take a look at the ideas given on these pages.

GUIDELINES
• Warm up for at least 5 minutes before you begin with light cardiovascular activities, such as walking or biking.
• Exercise on a firm, padded surface. Place a small pillow or folded towel under the head and neck when lying on your back, or under your hips and forehead when lying face down.
• During stretching exercises, breathe normally. Move into each position slowly and stretch only to the point of mild tension–not pain. Hold the stretch without bouncing or straining. Stretch daily, or at least every other day.
• Perform each strength and stabilization exercise at a slow pace to the point of moderate muscle fatigue. Breathe normally or exhale on the exertion phase of each exercise. Start with a few repetitions and gradually increase to 10 to 15 if possible. Stabilization and strength exercises should be done every other day for best results.
• During stabilization exercises, contract your abdominal muscles to maintain a neutral position of the pelvis. Keep the shoulders gently pulled back and down while keeping the nape of the neck long and the chin level.
• Avoid or modify the exercises that cause pain by decreasing the range of motion and/or the number of repetitions.
• In addition to performing this program regularly, it is important to participate in low- or non-impact cardiovascular activities such as walking, biking, or swimming.

The spa stretching regime
from the Golden Door, California

The following stretches have been designed by the fitness experts at The Golden Door. Not only will they help to lengthen and strengthen muscles, they are also designed to strengthen and increase the flexibility of the muscles of the spine and improve posture.

THE EXERCISES
Stretch: lower back
Lie on your back with your knees bent directly over your waistline. Hold behind the thighs and bring your knees towards your chest. The knees can be together or slightly apart. Hold for 15 to 30 seconds. Repeat 1 to 2 times.

Stretch: hip flexor
Lie on your back, place your hands behind one thigh, and pull towards your chest. Rotate each ankle 5 times in each direction. Keep the other leg straight and press the calf towards the floor. Hold for 15 to 30 seconds. Repeat 1 to 2 times.

Stretch: hip and buttocks
Lie on your back with your left foot on the floor and right ankle crossed over the left thigh. Press the right knee away from your body. Lift the left foot off the floor and bring the left thigh towards your chest. Reach through your legs and hold on to the back of the left thigh (a). Repeat on the other side. Hold for 15 to 30 seconds. Repeat 1 to 2 times for each leg.

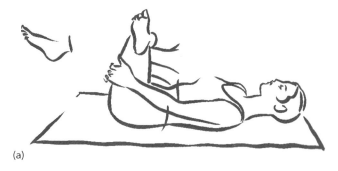

(a)

Stretch: side-lying quad

Lie on one side with your head cradled in your bottom arm and with the bottom leg slightly bent. Hold on to the top ankle and pull towards your buttocks while pressing your hips forward and keeping your leg parallel to the floor (b). Repeat on other leg. Hold for 15 to 30 seconds. Repeat 1 to 2 times.

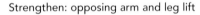

(b)

Stabilization: bridging

Lie on your back and with your feet a hip-width apart and knees bent 90 degrees, slowly raise your buttocks from the floor, keeping your abdominals tight and hips even. Lower one vertebra at a time. Repeat 5 to 10 times.

Strengthen: opposing arm and leg lift

Lie face down, arms overhead, palms down. Put a towel under your hips if necessary. Slowly raise your right arm and left leg, without twisting your hips or shoulders (d). Exhale. Return to the starting position and then work on the alternate sides. Pull in your abdominals and keep your neck and shoulders relaxed. Hold for 3 to 5 seconds. Repeat 10 to 15 times.

Stretch: abdominal curl

Lie on your back with your legs up on a chair (or with your knees bent and feet on the floor) and with your hands behind your head or across your chest. While keeping your head aligned with your spine, tighten your abdominals by lifting your shoulders off the floor (c). Repeat 5 to 10 times.

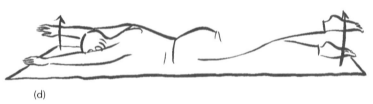

(d)

(c)

Strengthen: wall squat

With your head, shoulders, and hips against a wall, walk your feet away from the wall about 24 to 36 inches. Position your feet a hip-width apart, bend your knees to 45 degrees (work up to 90 degrees). Keep your knees aligned over your ankles, lift your toes off the floor, and hold the position. Hold for 20 to 60 seconds. Repeat 3 to 5 times.

Stretch: lower back and abdominals

Lie on your stomach with your legs straight and arms bent, with forearms and chest on the floor. Press up your torso while keeping your hips flat on the floor, head straight, and eyes looking forward (e). Hold for 5 seconds. Then return to the starting position. Repeat 3 to 5 times.

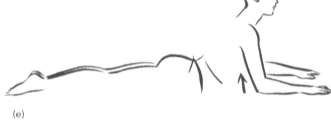

(e)

Hand-weight training

There is a very good reason to incorporate weight training into your fitness routine. After the age of twenty-five, you lose about half a pound of muscle every year. Worse still, if you don't exercise, fat replaces muscle. Not only does your shape begin to suffer but your strength decreases too. Add to this the fact that, as we age, the risk of osteoporosis increases, and the picture does not look good. Working out with weights, however, goes some way toward protecting against muscle loss and decreased bone density.

GUIDELINES

• Perform each exercise at a slow, controlled pace, on two to three non-consecutive days per week.
• Exhale on the difficult (exertion) part of the exercise, or breathe normally.
• Exercises for one of the large muscle groups (leg, back, and chest) should be performed before the smaller muscle groups (arms, calves).
• Follow the program in the order outlined.
• Complete the exercises for each muscle group before moving on to the next.
• Increase repetitions, weight, and/or sets gradually for continuous improvements. For general strength training, increase to next weight when you reach 12 repetitions comfortably. Use a chart to track your progress.
• Rest for 30 to 45 seconds between sets if using heavy weights (8 lb or more for women, 12 lb or more for men). For lighter weights, rest 20 to 30 seconds between sets.
• For all standing, upper-body exercises, stand with feet comfortably apart, knees relaxed, and hips tucked under.
• Perform each exercise through the full range of motion without snapping joints. Never compromise sound technique or good posture to finish a repetition.

The spa hand weight-training program
from Henlow Grange Health Farm, Bedfordshire, UK

WARM-UP EXERCISES
1. Warm up on a bike or treadmill or do any other rhythmical activity for at least 5 minutes.
2. Do shoulder rolls. Stand or sit with arms down at the sides. Circle shoulders forward 5 times and back 5 times.
3. Do arm circles. Perform slow, large arm circles with elbows slightly bent. Perform 5 forward and 5 back.
4. Do sky reaches. Stand with feet apart, knees relaxed, and pelvis tilted up. With arms overhead, reach alternate hands towards the ceiling, bending forward slightly at the waist. Perform 5 each side.
5. Do squats. With feet 40 to 48 inches apart and toes slightly turned out, slowly bend knees halfway, keeping heels flat on the floor and knees aligned over the ankles, then straighten. Perform 5 to 10 times.
6. Stretch the muscles that are going to be used, holding each stretch for 8 to 10 seconds.

WEIGHT TRAINING EXERCISES
Legs: squats
Stand with your feet hip-width apart, toes forward, arms straight at sides, hands grasping weights. Bend your legs halfway, keeping your back straight. Flexing at the hips, lean forward slightly and imagine that you are sitting in a chair with your heels down on the ground.

Legs: heel raises
Stand with your feet slightly apart, with your arms straight at your sides, and hands grasping weights. Perform the exercise from the following three foot positions: toes forward, toes out, toes in. Keeping your legs straight, lift your heels off the floor. Rise onto your toes then lower your heels.

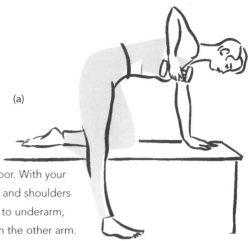

(a)

Back: single-arm row

Place your left hand and left knee on a bench and keep your right foot on the floor. With your right arm straight, grasp a weight in your right hand. Keeping your back straight and shoulders square, bend your right elbow, aiming it toward the ceiling, bring the weight up to underarm, and squeeze the shoulder blade (a). Do not twist your back. Repeat exercise with the other arm.

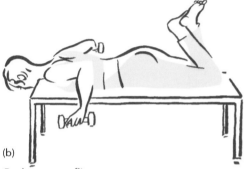

(b)

Back: reverse flies

Lie face down on a bench, elbows slightly bent. Grasp the weights below the bench, palms facing inward. Lift the weights out to the sides at shoulder level while squeezing your shoulder blades together (b).

Chest: bench press

Lie back on a bench, knees bent, feet flat on the bench, and elbows bent at shoulder level. Hold the weights at shoulder height, palms facing knees. Keeping your arms shoulder-width apart, press the weights towards the ceiling and straighten your arms above your chest (d). Avoid locking your elbows.

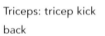

(d)

Shoulders: shoulder press

Sit or stand upright with your legs apart. Hold the weights above your shoulders with palms facing forward. Elbows should point outward. Straightening your arms, lift the weights over your head alongside your ears.

Shoulders: upright row

Stand with your legs apart. Grasp the weights in front of your thighs with your palms facing the thighs. Bend your elbows while lifting the weights to your chin. Attempt to lift your elbows higher than the weights.

Triceps: tricep kick back

Stand or sit upright with your elbows pulled backward at your sides. Hold the weights next to your chest, palms facing each other. Straighten your arms, pushing the weights back (c). Keep your elbows pulled into your sides.

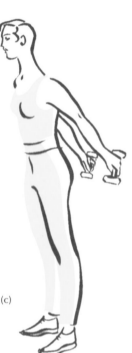

(c)

Biceps: pull-ups

Stand or sit upright with your elbows pulled into your sides. Hold the weights in front of your thighs with your palms facing forward. Keeping your elbows at your side, bend your arms and pull the weights up to your shoulders, and then slowly lower them back to your thighs. For variation, alternate your arms or perform the exercise with your palms facing inward.

Waist: side bends

Stand with your feet apart, arms relaxed, and pelvis tilted up. Allow your arms to hang straight down at your sides with hands grasping the weights, and palms facing your thighs. Slowly bend from your waist to the left side, lifting your right hand to your underarm while bending your right elbow. Then slowly repeat on the other side. Avoid bending over or arching your back.

Walking back to fitness

Even if you can't get to a gym, walking is one of the most effective ways of getting back into shape. It has also become one of the most popular activities at spas because it is so easy to take home and fit into your everyday life. From a gentle hike to a brisk walk, you can choose the style that suits your needs and vary it as you desire. At the Golden Door, the morning hike is one of the most exhilarating ways you could wish to start the day. After a week of morning hikes and brisk walks at the spa, I came home feeling fit enough to enter the next Olympics . . . well almost. And even if you don't live in such beautiful surroundings, you can find a local park or head for the countryside on weekends to get your walking fix.

The most natural form of exercise, done on a regular basis, walking can lower the risk of cardiovascular disease and osteoporosis, reduce body fat, tone muscle, and increase overall stamina. Not only that, but because it is low impact, risk of injury is also low. You also need little in the way of equipment so you can exercise wherever you go.

The spa walking program

WARM-UP
Always warm up with a three-minute slow walk followed by some light stretching, if needed. Drink water before, during, and after walking.

GUIDELINES
• Avoid a bouncy, bobbing motion when you walk.
• When walking uphill, take smaller steps and maintain good alignment.
• Take smaller steps when walking downhill. Soften knees to decrease impact.
• Progress gradually.

WALKING TECHNIQUES
Basic walking (strolling up to 3.5 miles per hour)
• Keep head straight with chin parallel to the ground and eyes looking ahead.
• Keep shoulders down, back, and relaxed, and chest lifted.
• Keep pelvis in neutral position while lengthening torso. Hands and arms should be relaxed and moving in opposition to the legs in a long pendulum swing close to the body. Avoid crossing the midline of the body.
• Land on the heel and roll through the ball of the foot.
• Stride length is determined by your leg length, muscle tightness, and degree of pelvic rotation.

Fitness walking (3.6 to 5 miles per hour)
• Maintain good posture as in Basic Walking, but with a slight forward lean from the ankles.
• Keep elbows bent at about 90 degrees. Avoid crossing the midline of the body with the hands and do not swing the hands higher than the top of chest. On the back swing, bring elbow slightly behind the body, and hand to the front of the hip. Keep hands relaxed.
• Keep elbows close to the body. Movement of the arms is produced at the shoulders, not the elbows.
• Speed up arm swing to increase walking speed.
• Land mid-heel with the forefoot raised. Roll from heel to the ball of the foot. The knees are almost fully extended but do not lock. Hips should rotate slightly–this is a natural motion.

Modified race walking (5 miles per hour plus)
• Maintain the same posture as Fitness Walking. Increase speed of arms and legs.
• Hands should not reach further back than the buttocks on the back swing.
• Walk with feet closer together. This results in a natural hip rotation.
• Keep ball of rear foot on ground until the heel of the forward foot has contacted the ground.
• Avoid hyper-extending the knee joint.

COOL DOWN

Always cool down for 3 to 5 minutes, then perform some of these static stretches.

STATIC STRETCHES

Waist and upper back

With one hand on your hip, reach the other arm over your head while bending to the opposite side from the waist. Keep hips still. Hold for 10 to 30 seconds. Perform 1 to 2 times on each side.

Chest and front shoulder

Stand with your feet shoulder-width apart. Clasp your hands behind your back with the palms inwards. Press your hands down toward the floor, bringing your shoulders down and back at the same time (a). Hold for 10 to 30 seconds. Perform 1 to 2 times.

(a)

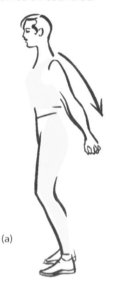

Hip and back

Stand tall. Grasp your left thigh with your left hand and bring the top of the thigh toward your chest. Place the right hand against a wall for support. Circle the raised ankle 5 times inward, then 5 times outward. Switch sides.

Front thigh (quadriceps)

Bend your right knee, and with your right hand grab hold of your right ankle and bring your heel toward your buttocks, keeping your opposite hand on a wall for stability if necessary. Keep your knees close together, hips pressed forward, and body upright. Hold for 10 to 30 seconds. Perform 1 to 2 times on each leg.

Rear thigh (hamstring)

Stand with one heel on the ground or elevated on a step with the leg straight and the other leg 2 to 3 feet away from the step, knee bent. Press your hips backwards while keeping your back straight (b). Hold for 10 to 30 seconds. Perform 1 to 2 times on each leg.

Calf (calf stretch)   (b)

Step forward, bend your front knee, and press your heel to the floor. Keep your back leg straight and toe pointing forward. Then bring your rear foot slightly closer to your front foot and bend the back knee while keeping your heels down and body weight over the rear foot. Hold for 10 to 30 seconds in each position. Perform 1 time on each leg.

WHAT TO LOOK FOR IN A WALKING SHOE

1. low cut
2. beveled heel
3. Achilles notch
4. flexible forefoot
5. light weight
6. roomy toe box
7. good heel stability
8. adequate cushioning

SPA face
AND body blitz

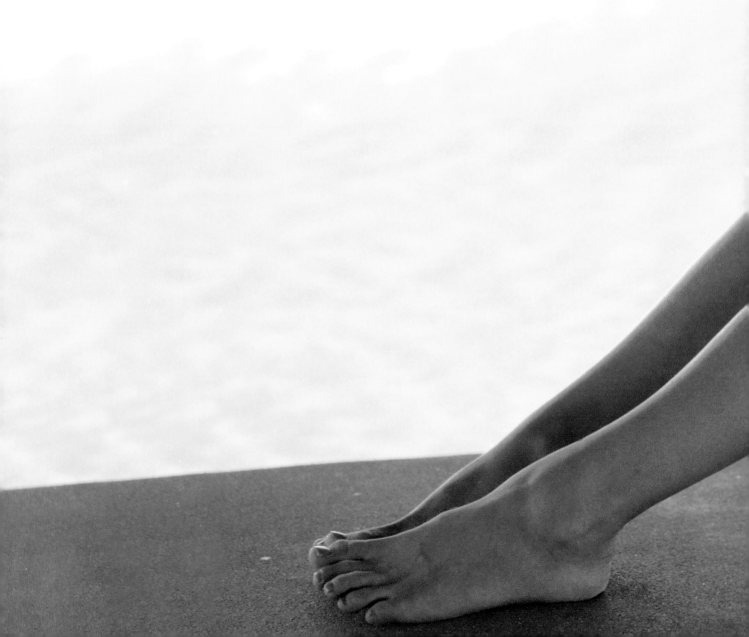

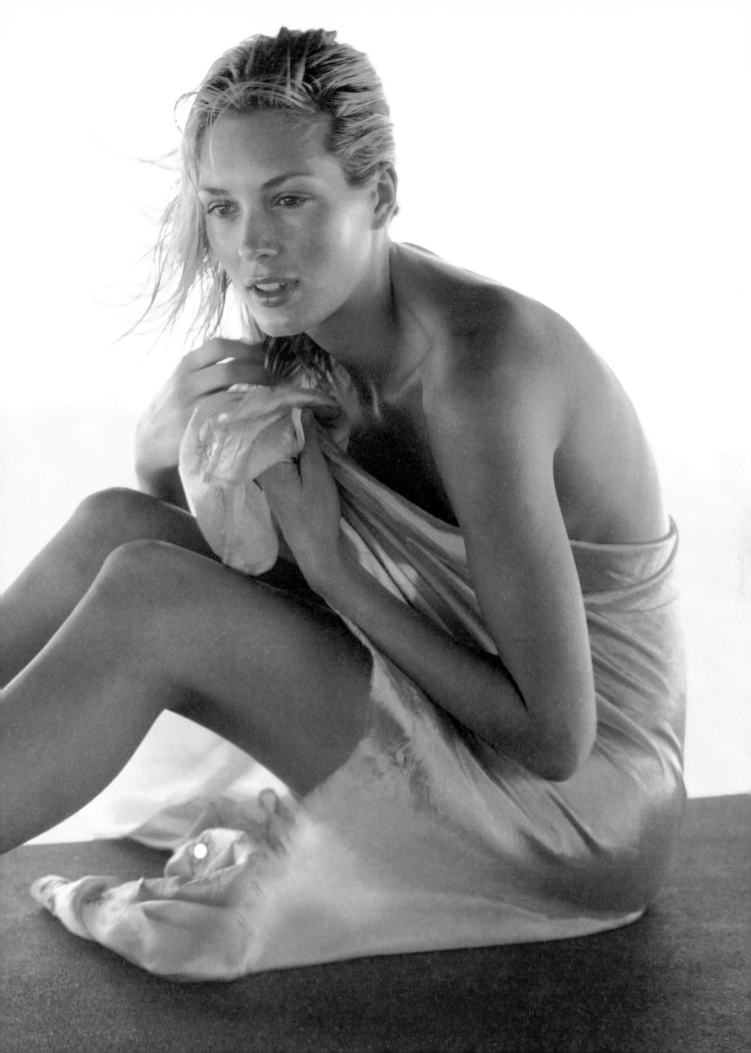

Body buffing

Exfoliating, sloughing, polishing–call it what you will. Although our skin naturally renews itself every twenty-eight or so days and sheds any dead skin cells naturally, it always benefits from a helping hand. One of the most instantly gratifying spa and salon treatments, body buffing not only leaves skin smooth-as-a-baby, but helps to rev up circulation and stimulate the lymphatic system– the body's natural waste disposal unit. While it's a blissful treat to have this done for you, it is equally rewarding at home. We have gathered some of the best body polishing recipes and techniques from spas around the globe.

Native body glow

Boost circulation with this remineralizing and refreshing scrub from Vista Clara Ranch Resort and Spa in New Mexico. It uses traditional Native American ingredients.

1 cup Dead Sea salts (available at health food shops and pharmacies)
1/2 cup wholewheat flour
1/2 cup carrier oil such as almond oil
5 drops sage or cedarwood essential oil

1. Mix the ingredients in a small bowl set beside your bathtub. Shower to dampen your skin and apply the mixture to your entire body, working on one section at a time.
2. Massage gently on freshly shaved areas and more vigorously on rough spots, such as elbows, knees, and feet. Don't leave on your skin for more than 5 minutes.
3. Rinse thoroughly. The result? Super-smooth, soft skin. Do not repeat this scrub more than two times weekly.

Salt body scrub

Pep up circulation and buff skin with this invigorating body polish that comes from Lake Austin Resort in Texas.

30 drops essential oil of lavender or rosemary
1/2 cup vegetable oil
1/2 cup Dead Sea salts

1. In a bowl, mix the essential oil with the vegetable oil and then add the Dead Sea salts. Blend thoroughly. Choose lavender essential oil for a relaxing blend or rosemary essential oil for a refreshing mix.
2. Use the mixture to scrub and exfoliate the body, ensuring that your skin is pre-showered and still damp. Work upwards from the ankles. Rinse and pat skin dry gently. The result? Tingling, refreshed skin.

Coconut body glow

This gentle body scrub from The Mandara Spa at The Chedi, Bali, Indonesia, is perfect for delicate skin as it exfoliates effectively but without causing irritation.

1/2 coconut, grated
1/4 tsp turmeric powder or freshly grated turmeric root
8 oz carrots, grated
2 tbsp gelatin powder

1. Mix the freshly grated coconut with the turmeric and gently rub over damp skin. Leave on for 5 minutes, then wipe off with a warm cloth.
2. Mix the carrot and gelatin together and apply to the skin. Leave for a few minutes then rinse off. The result? Skin feels smoother and moister.

Body polish

This exotic body scrub, created by spa beauty company Li'Tya for Daintree Eco-Lodge and Spa, Queensland, Australia, includes indigenous ingredients.

4 tbsp natural yogurt
12 macadamia nuts, finely ground
2 tbsp elder flowers, ground (available at health food stores)
4 eucalyptus leaves, finely chopped (or 8 drops eucalyptus essential oil)

1. Combine the natural yogurt, finely ground macadamia nuts, ground elder flowers, and finely chopped eucalyptus leaves or essential oil.
2. Rub into your body, massaging well to ensure full absorption. Wipe your skin clean with a warm, damp cloth. The result? Smoother, cleaner skin.

Oriental body glow

Stimulate your circulation and soften your skin with this traditional Thai body scrub recipe from the Banyan Tree Spa in Phuket, Thailand.

1 cup liquid honey
1/2 cup sesame seeds
1 tsp dried herbs, such as mint or lavender leaf

1. Blend the ingredients.
2. Massage it into your skin from face to toe, working slowly and steadily so that your skin tingles. Finish by showering with warm water. The result? Gorgeously caramel-scented skin that is satiny-smooth.

Bali kopi scrub

For one of the most unusual sensory experiences, try this skin-smoothing exfoliant, found at many of the premier Far Eastern spas, such as The Mandara Spas in Malaysia, and The Chedi, The Ibah, Bali Padma, and Nikko in Bali.

7 oz coffee beans, ground
3 tbsp kaolin clay (available at health food stores and pharmacies)
1/4 tsp of ground pumice stone (optional)
8 oz carrots, grated
1 tsp gelatin, already set (optional)
water

1. Grind the coffee beans finely and mix with the kaolin clay and ground pumice, if using. Add enough water to make a paste.
2. Rub over damp skin, allow to dry for a few minutes, then rub off vigorously.
3. Follow by rubbing in the carrots mixed with the gelatin (if using), which acts as a moisture replenisher. Shower and pat skin dry. The result? Amazingly silky skin, deliciously scented with the aroma of coffee.

Soothing baths

Now part and parcel of most spa beauty programs, aromatherapy has been used by many ancient cultures as part of well-being rituals. In aromatherapy, essential oils extracted from flowers and plants are used in massage, inhalation, and bathing to benefit mind, body, and spirit. When using them in the bath, stick to the recommended doses as they are very potent.

Herbal baths and treatments have become more popular at conventional spas and can now be found on most menus. For home treatments, herbs can be purchased from a wide number of health food stores (see home-spa suppliers, page 140). As with essential oils, seek medical advice before using them, especially orally.

You can use herbs to make tisanes and infusions to drink and for the bath. When you are using them in the bath, put the loose herbs in a muslin bag (available from most health food stores) or simply place a handful in the middle of a muslin cloth square and tie the corners at the top to prevent herbs escaping. Place the bag under the hot tap as you run the bath or leave to steep for a few minutes before you get in.

GUIDELINES
• If you do suffer from any serious medical condition or are pregnant, consult your doctor or midwife before using essential oils.
• Although there are a huge number of inexpensive oils available on the street and in supermarkets, you get what you pay for when it comes to essential oils (see stockists for suggested reputable suppliers).

Desert journey bath tea

Evocative of the tranquility and aromas of the southwest, this luxurious bath treat from Westward Look Resort, Arizona, USA, is guaranteed to leave you feeling calm and at one with nature. The Desert Journey Bath Tea itself is available direct from the spa (see directory) or you can make a similar recipe as follows.

1 tbsp each of rose petals, citrus peel, lavender, rosemary, chamomile and sage
10 drops lavender essential oil

1. Add the lavender to the herbs and store in a glass jar, preferably dark glass. If you can't find a dark glass jar, store in a clear glass container away from the light.
2. Shake to mix thoroughly and add 2 heaping tablespoons to a muslin bag or piece of cloth tied with string. Steep for a few minutes in a comfortably warm bath, light some candles, and put on some soothing music. Westward Look's spa director, Lydia Corona, suggests listening to some Native American flute music—check out anything by R. Carlos Nakai (see page 23).

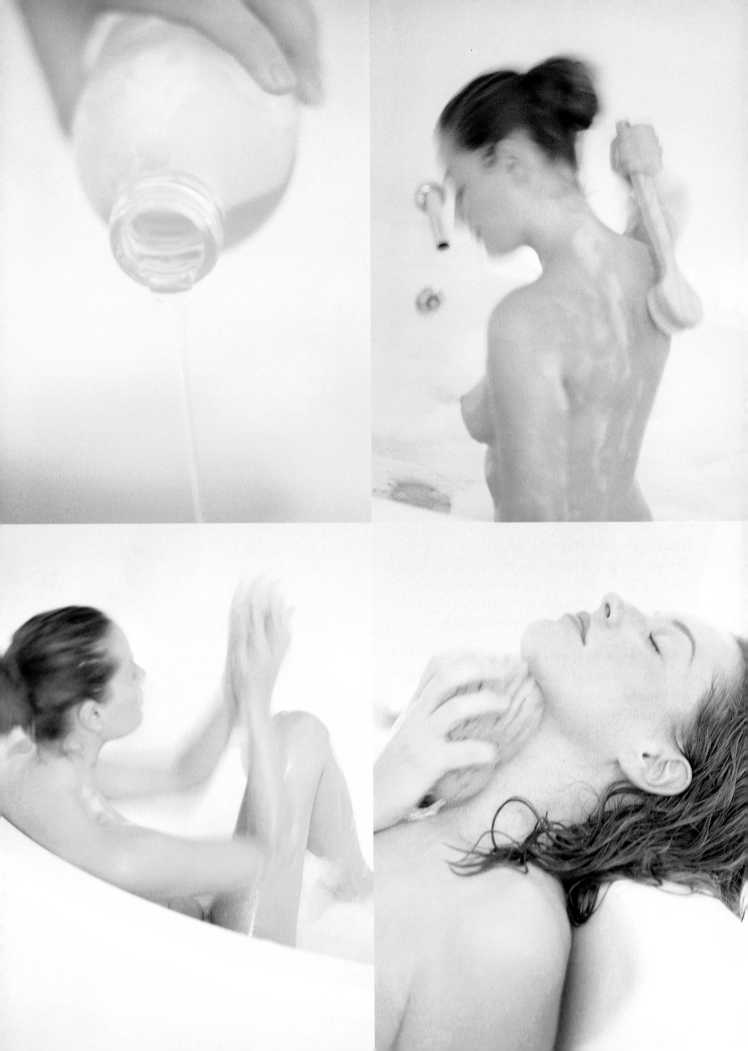

Restorative herbal bath

For a luxurious soak, try this herbal bath from The Spa at The Hyatt Regency-Coolum in Queensland, Australia.

herbal bag (see below for recipe)
Coral Moon bath oils (see below for recipes)
cold eucalyptus-fragranced towel
rolled towel for head

1. Fill your bath with warm water and, while the bath is running, add the bag of herbs. Choose your oil combination depending on your mood (see below) and add to the bath water. Light some candles, turn on your most relaxing music, and settle into the bath. Soak for 30 minutes.

RESTORATIVE HERBAL BAG

2 tablespoons each of lemon balm, lemon verbena, citronella grass, marigold flowers, geranium flowers, mint leaves and ½ cup of oats. Place in a glass jar to store. Add a handful to a muslin bag or cloth and steep in warm bath water.

CORAL MOON BATH OILS

Tension and stress relieving blend: In a cup, mix 4 drops each of geranium, clary sage, rose, and frankincense essential oils.
Relaxing blend: In a cup, mix 4 drops each of chamomile, lavender, orange, and petitgrain essential oils.
Refreshing blend: In a cup, mix 4 drops each of peppermint, lemon, and bergamot essential oils.

Cleansing bath

To detoxify mind and body, try this cleansing bath, inspired by the detoxifying aromatherapy baths offered at many Asian spas.

ginger, sage, and rosemary essential oils
1 tbsp almond or jojoba oil

1. Add 3 drops each of the essential oils to a warm bath, just before you step into the bath. Inhale deeply, lie back, and soak for 20 minutes.
2. Dry your skin thoroughly and then massage the same combination of oils blended with the almond or jojoba oil into your skin. Wrap up in a warm terry cloth robe and climb into bed. Rest for at least half an hour.
3. To complete the process, drink 6 to 8 glasses of water throughout the day or, if you are going straight to bed, sip a cup of fennel herbal tea.

Hot aroma bath soak

For a soothing bath, try this recipe from the Golden Door in California, created by Cindy Fitzgerald from the spa's beauty department.

Choose your favorite flower, be it roses, gardenias, or lavender, and put two cupfuls of dried flowers into a cheesecloth and allow to steep for a few minutes in a hot tub. Once infused, step in and soak for at least 20 minutes.

Thalassotherapy treat

The basis of many curative programs at European and Japanese spas, thalassotherapy uses the healing power of water. In thalassotherapy (from the Greek "thalassa," meaning "sea"), sea water and marine extracts are used in a variety of treatments from underwater massage to body wraps. The first modern thalassotherapy center was set up by Dr. Rene Bagot at Roscoff in Brittany, France, and since then, centers have been set up along the French coast at locations such as Deauville and Quiberon and on the African Atlantic at Casablanca. Bagot discovered that the minerals and trace elements present in sea water were almost identical to those found in our own blood plasma. By heating up the sea water, our bodies can absorb these minerals by osmosis.

Inspired by the sea water and seaweed enriched baths at the Hotel Miramar's Institute of Thalassotherapy Louison Bobet, Biarritz, France, this restorative soak will boost flagging energy levels and help to detoxify.

1 cup dried or micronized seaweed
1/2 cup very hot water
3 drops lavender essential oil

1. Dissolve the dried or micronized seaweed (available from health food stores, spas, and beauty salons) in the very hot water and add to a bath heated to 100°F.
2. Add the lavender essential oil just before you step in and soak for at least 20 minutes. Wrap up warmly after you dry yourself and try to drink as much water as possible to aid the elimination process.

Therapeutic bath

For a restorative spa bath, similar to those found at the spa at Baden in Austria, ensure that water is between 96 and 100°F to aid relaxation. Shower first with warm water, then run a warm bath. To soothe frazzled nerves, add a handful of valerian; to ease tension, try chamomile; and to stimulate sluggish circulation, add rosemary. Place the herbs in muslin or cheesecloth and tie with string. Dunk in the water and allow to steep for at least 5 minutes before you get in. While your bath is running, take a handful of damp sea salt (see Body Buffing recipes, page 86) blended with a little oil and massage into your skin. Slip into the bath and soak for at least 20 minutes.

Refreshing sitz bath

One of the staples at Austrian, German, and Hungarian spas, sitz baths help to promote restful sleep, encourage relaxation, and stimulate circulation and digestion. Fill your bath with enough warm water to allow you to sit in the tub with the water level with your waist. Add 6 to 8 drops of a refreshing essential oil such as mandarin, tangerine, lemon balm, or peppermint, wrap your torso in a warm towel and soak for about 10 minutes. Finish with a cool head-to-toe shower.

Power shower

If you have a high-pressure shower at home, try this invigorating hydrotherapy treatment based on a treatment at the Blitzguss spa. Take a warm shower first, then switch to cold water and spray areas prone to poor circulation and cellulite such as thighs, buttocks, hips, and upper arms, for 20 seconds at a time. Switch back to warm water for 1 or 2 minutes, then back to cold for a final spritz. Work your way up the body, starting with your legs. For a general tonic and immune-system boost, use the same technique to spray your whole body, starting with your face, then moving on to arms, chest, stomach, back, buttocks, legs, and feet. Finish with a brisk rub with a sisal mitt, and pat skin dry with a fluffy towel.

Body wraps and packs

Body wraps, mud packs, and masks come in a variety of guises. From the exotic experience of a rose oil body or papaya wrap to the deep-cleansing benefits of a seaweed, kaolin, or fuller's earth pack, there's a recipe for every skin requirement. You can adapt the recipes to suit your own personal preferences and needs, adding a little honey for extra moisture or specific essential oils to treat problem zones. With endless possibilities, you'll never get bored. To get you started, try these restorative wraps and packs, available at some of the world's foremost spas.

Aromatic body pack

This deep cleansing earth pack is similar to body packs available at many Middle Eastern and Asian spas. Particularly recommended for problem skin and those suffering from blemished backs, the clay or fuller's earth helps to absorb impurities and promote healing.

1½ cups green clay or fuller's earth (available from health food stores and pharmacies)
1 cup water
2 tbsp organic clear honey
2 drops frankincense essential oil
2 drops vetiver essential oil
4 drops lavender or rose essential oil

1. Mix the clay or fuller's earth with the water and blend into a smooth paste.
2. Add the honey and essential oils and apply to required areas. Leave on for 15 minutes, then shower off with warm water. Pat the skin dry.

Essential rose body wrap

Indulge in this nourishing and deliciously scented body treatment originating from the Lake Austin Spa Resort in Texas. At the spa, skin is exfoliated with ground olive stones, then smothered in organic essential oil of rose, and wrapped in layers of thermal blankets. Finally, frankincense and rose essential oils are massaged into the skin for gentle stimulation of blood flow and lymphatic circulation. The result? Removal of dead cells and dry skin, improvement in skin tone and texture, and a feeling of being rested, calmed, and deeply relaxed.

body scrub (see pages 86–7 for recipes)
½ cup carrier oil, such as almond, avocado, or jojoba oil
rose essential oil
plastic sheet
warm blankets
hot-water bottle
frankincense essential oil

1. Exfoliate your skin with a body scrub and shower off with warm water. Pat skin dry.
2. Add the rose oil to ½ cup of carrier oil and smooth on to your skin from face to toe. Save the leftover oil for the next step of the treatment. Wrap up in a plastic sheet and blankets and have a hot-water bottle at your feet. Lie down and relax for 15 to 20 minutes.
3. Add the frankincense oil to the leftover rose and carrier oil blend. Finish your relaxing treat by massaging your body with the oil and leave it to soak in before dressing.

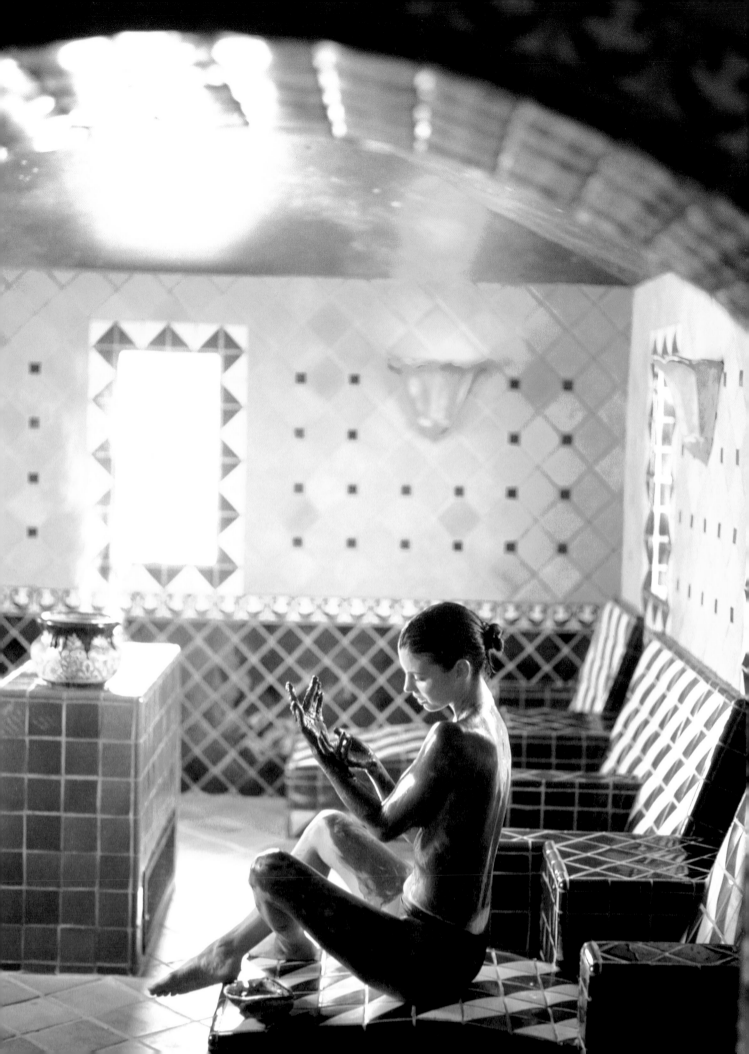

Aloe and lavender wrap

This has to be one of the most skin-soothing treatments available, East or West. Adapted from a recipe from The Jimbaran Spa at The Four Seasons Resort in Bali, this will take your skin from dehydrated to deliciously moisturized. At the Jimbaran, the treatment also involves using banana leaves but as these are not too easy to come by, use a cotton sarong or sheet instead.

1 tsp fresh aloe pulp (plants are available from most garden centers and florists)
10 tbsp aloe vera gel (available from health food stores)
lavender essential oil
1/2 cup distilled water
juice of 4 lemons or limes
2 cups warm water
body lotion

1. Mix the fresh aloe with the aloe vera gel and apply to your body.
2. Add 10 drops of the lavender oil to the distilled water and pour into an atomizer, and spray all over your body.
3. Lie down and place a cotton sarong or sheet gently over you. Relax for about 20 minutes.
4. Add the lemon or lime juice to the 2 cups of warm water. Also add 4 drops of the lavender essential oil. Shower with warm water, then splash your body with the lemon or lime juice water.
5. Rinse again with warm water, pat your skin dry, and then massage in a generous amount of your favorite body lotion.

Papaya body mask

A legendary body treat at Far Eastern spas, including The Oriental Spa in Bangkok, Thailand, papaya contains papain, an enzyme that helps to soften skin and aid digestion. It is also a natural source of AHAs (alpha hydroxy acids), which help to exfoliate the skin.

2 ripe papayas
2 drops mandarin essential oil
2 drops vetiver

1. Blend the ripe papayas in a food processor until smooth, then add the mandarin essential oil and vetiver.
2. Apply to your body and wrap up in a plastic sheet for 20 minutes. Rinse off with warm water.

Body mud

This purifying body mask is a favorite at Daintree Eco-Lodge and Spa in Queensland, Australia.

1 tsp dried seaweed
1 cup water
2 tbsp kaolin clay
1 tbsp rose water
2 tbsp macadamia oil
1 tbsp clear organic honey
1 drop peppermint essential oil
2 drops sandalwood essential oil
1 drop lavender essential oil
1 drop sage essential oil

1. Boil the dried seaweed in the water for 5 minutes and then leave to cool.
2. Combine the kaolin, rose water, and macadamia oil with the honey. Add the peppermint, sandalwood, lavender, and sage essential oils and combine thoroughly.
3. Smoothe over your body. Keep your body wrapped or warm for 10 to 15 minutes and then rinse off with warm water.

Detox

If the word detox sends shivers down your spine, listen up. When it comes to an instant body overhaul, a detox cannot only be satisfying but a pleasurable ritual. Created by the experts at The Spa at St. David's Hotel, Cardiff, UK, try the detox routine given below, guaranteed to sweep away any cobwebs, uplift your spirits, boost your energy levels, and leave you feeling ultra-clean.

DETOX ROUTINE

Step 1: Brush skin

Using light, upward movements, stroke your skin with a sisal body brush or hemp mitt, always working toward the heart. Stroke each part of the body three times, working from the soles of your feet upward. Body brushing helps to stimulate the body's lymphatic system, reducing fluid retention and, some experts believe, cellulite.

Step 2: Shower

Put 3 to 4 drops of peppermint essential oil on to a sisal pad or hemp mitt. Massage this into your skin as you shower in comfortably warm water. Work upwards from the ankles, using small, brisk, circular movements.

Step 3: Exfoliate

Use a handful of sea salt mixed with a tablespoon of body oil to buff damp skin. Use circular movements, working from the feet upward. Pat the skin dry and wrap up warmly in a terry cloth robe or loose clothing.

Daintree body brush

For an invigorating, detoxifying experience, try this body brushing routine from Daintree Eco-Lodge and Spa in Queensland, Australia. Not only does it help to remove dead skin cells but it also stimulates blood circulation. Ideally, body brushing should be done every morning before showering or bathing.

• Using a body brush on your legs, stoke upward toward the heart, following with your free hand.
• Use the same method on the arms.
• Stroke the back, three movements on the right side, then the middle, and then on the left side. (You may need assistance!)
• Use fast, upward movements on the buttocks to get the blood flowing. (It's great for cellulite.)
• Use circular, clockwise strokes on the stomach.
• Then shower or soak in a warm bath. Moisturize the body with your favorite lotion or oil.

Deep cleansing body rub

Cleanse and detoxify skin with this stimulating rub, inspired by traditional Far Eastern spa recipes.

2 tbsp ground sandalwood powder
4 tbsp goat's milk yogurt
2 tsp honey

1. Mix the ground sandalwood powder with the goat's milk yogurt and honey and massage vigorously into damp skin.
2. Leave on for 15 to 20 minutes, then rinse off with warm water. The result is glowing, fresh-looking skin.

Deluxe body treats

There are some spa body recipes that deserve to be dubbed deluxe. Here are a few of my own favorite indulgences, from the sublime Petals body treatment at Ojai Valley Inn and Spa, California, which makes you feel like you're in heaven, to the delectable vinotherapie from the Caudalie Institut in France. Prepare to experience Nirvana.

Petals

The signature body treatment at the Ojai Spa is one of life's most delicious pampering experiences. Based on soothing, nurturing essential rose oils known for their calming, romantic, and healing effects, Petals comprises three parts: exfoliation, showering, and moisturizing. At the Ojai Spa, Jurlique products are used, but you can substitute any good quality rose oils.

¼ cup corn starch
¼ cup corn meal
20 drops rose geranium essential oil
12 drops rose absolute essential oil
shower gel
rose essential oil
body lotion or massage oil

1. Begin by exfoliating the skin with a mixture of the corn starch, corn meal, rose geranium essential oil, and rose absolute essential oil. Combine all the ingredients and place in a shaker jar (like a sugar shaker with wide holes in the lid).
2. Sprinkle on the skin and gently exfoliate to remove the dead cells from the surface of the skin.
3. Shower in warm but not too hot water with a shower gel to which you have added 10 drops of rose essential oil.
4. Finally, smooth on a lotion or massage oil containing rose essential oil. Let the oil remain on the skin for at least a few hours. The effect is amazing: your skin will feel satiny soft and you will smell divine.

Vinotherapie body treat

At the Caudalie Institut de Vinotherapie, Martillac, France, treatments are based on grapes and wine. Both are rich sources of antioxidant polyphenols. Try this "at home" body treatment using the Caudalie Vinotherapie philosophy.

20 fresh grapes
5 tsp organic honey
10 tsp body scrub (see Body Buffing section, page 86)
grapeseed oil
vetiver or petitgrain essential oil

Blend the grapes with the honey and body scrub to make a paste. Massage it into damp skin and shower off. Pat your skin dry and finish by massaging your body from head to toe with grapeseed oil to which you have added vetiver or petitgrain essential oil.

Agua milk and honey

This is my all-time favorite indulgence, based on an ancient ayurvedic recipe by spa creators Rita Shrager and Leila Fazel, responsible for Agua at Delano in Florida, and, more recently, Agua at Sanderson in London.

4 tbsp powdered milk
3 tbsp organic clear honey
1 tbsp sesame oil

1. Combine the powdered milk with enough hot water to create a thin, smooth paste.
2. Combine the honey and sesame oil and heat gently in a double boiler or microwave until warm.
3. Apply the honey and oil mixture to as much of your body as possible using a sweeping massage movement. Lie down on a towel or cotton sheet and leave on for 10 minutes.
4. Remove the honey and oil mixture with the warm milk paste and a washcloth. The milk not only helps the sticky honey to glide off, but is excellent nourishment for the skin.

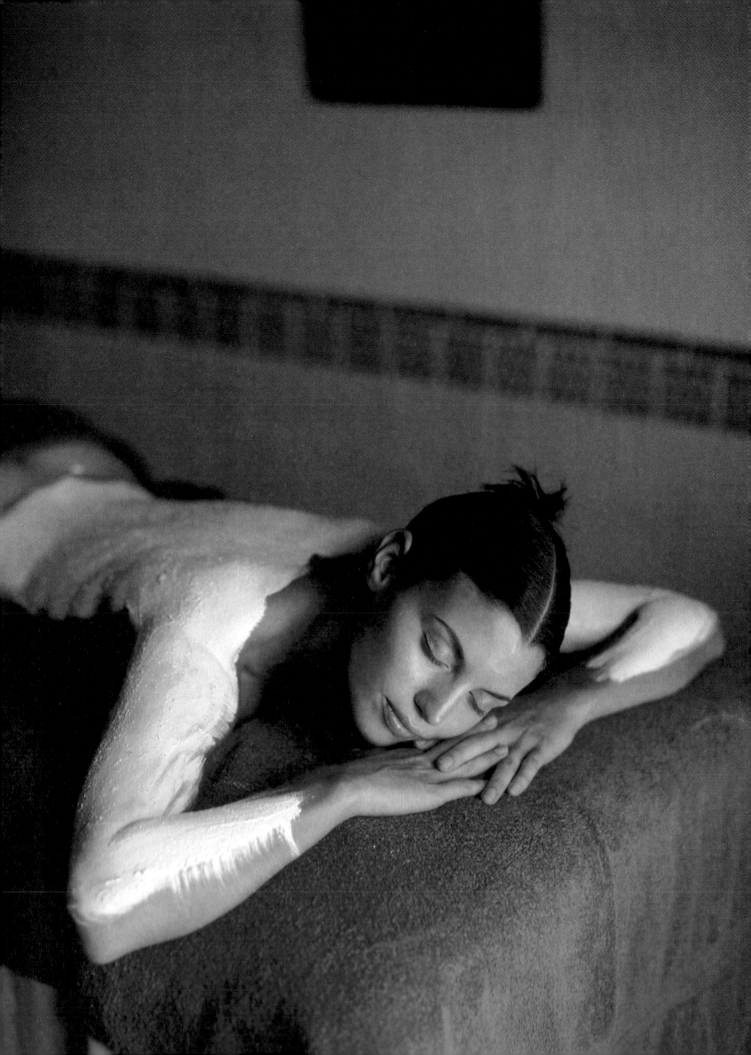

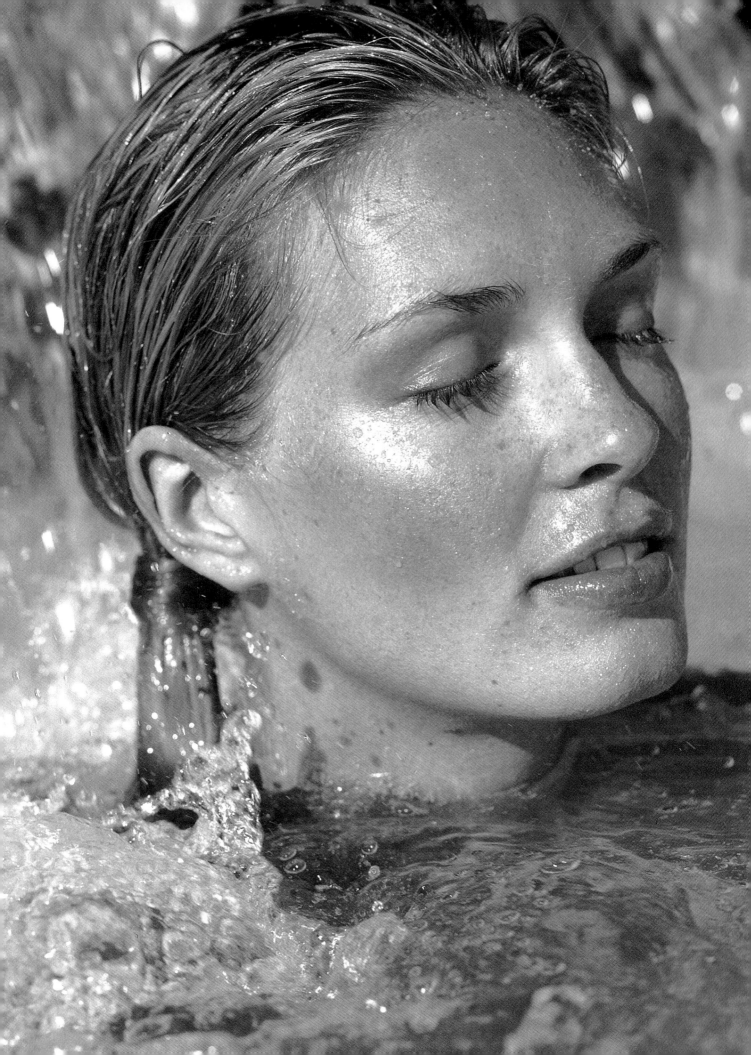

Spa treats for your face

While the focus of most spas is inner rather than outer beauty, no matter where they happen to be located across the globe, the majority of modern spas offer a mind-boggling array of facial pampering. Masks, scrubs, massage, and skin boosters, spa menus boast a host of beautifying treatments designed to restore our complexions to their former glory.

While there is no doubt that having a facial is one of the most wonderfully soothing therapies, you can reap some of the benefits of spa beauty wisdom at home. From traditional Malaysian and Balinese preparations to replenishing masks and scrubs from as far afield as Australia and Arizona, skin maintenance need never be mundane again. And if you are pushed for time, there are fast-track treats included on these pages from a 5-minute face mask to a 10-minute Shiatsu massage so that even when time is tight, you can still look groomed and feel pampered.

FACIAL MASSAGE
Nothing boosts circulation better than a facial massage. The basis of many spa facials, massage is key when it comes to maintaining skin tone as we age. For a once-a-week treat, use the following routine on freshly cleansed skin. Always use an oil when you massage to avoid dragging your skin and to allow your fingertips to move easily over your face and neck.

1. Choose a massage oil to suit your current skin type (see Facial Oils, this page; Essential Oils, page 100). You can add three to four different essential oils to your chosen carrier oil. Start by warming a teaspoon of oil in your palms. Rub your hands together briskly, then press them over your face, starting at your forehead and working your way outward and upward with firm pressure.

2. Next, use your fingertips to lightly tap all around your face. Start by tapping around your brows, underneath your eyes, along your cheekbones, under your nose, around your mouth, and along your jaw, always starting from the center of your face and working outward.
3. Add a little more oil to your palms, rub your palms together, and use your fingertips to massage your face with small circular motions, again starting at your brows, working around your eye sockets, across the cheekbones to your ears, and so on.
4. Add more oil and work from the base of your neck upwards to your chin and jaw line, using your fingers in sweeping motions.
5. Finish by pressing your palms and heels of your hands across your face, as in step 1.

FACIAL OILS
The following oils can be used to dilute essential oils for facial massage. Use 2 tablespoons of carrier oil to 10 drops of essential oil.

Apricot kernel oil: Perfect for use on the face as it is light in texture and easily absorbed. Skin type: suits all skin types, but particularly good for dry skin.
Avocado oil: Rich in vitamins A and B. Skin type: suitable for dry and sensitive skins.
Grapeseed oil: Rich in antioxidants, light in texture, and easily absorbed. Skin type: suits oily to combination skins.
Jojoba oil: A very versatile, balancing oil. Skin type: can be used to treat psoriasis and eczema and works equally well on oily or acne-prone skins.
Sweet almond oil: One of the most widely used skin softeners. Skin type: great for all skin types.
Vitamin E oil: Rich in anti-aging antioxidants. Skin type: excellent for very dry, skin and skin that needs a boost.

ESSENTIAL OILS

Always use a carrier or base oil when using essential oils, particularly on your face. Lavender and tea tree oil can be dabbed directly on to blemishes undiluted but those with sensitive skin should be very cautious.

Bergamot: An antiseptic and astringent, bergamot works to rebalance any oily and blemished skin.

Chamomile: Chamomile contains an ingredient called azulene that is known to be soothing and antibacterial.

Frankincense: It is excellent for very dry or mature skins, and it is incredibly soothing.

Jasmine: Suitable for most skin types, jasmine is a wonderful soother.

Lavender: It can be dabbed on to blemishes as it has antibacterial and antiseptic properties.

Patchouli: An effective moisturizer for very dry skin, it is also an antiseptic.

Rose: It works for all skin types and has an antibacterial action.

Sandalwood: Use it to treat acne-prone skin and to rebalance very oily complexions.

Tea tree: An excellent antiseptic with skin-healing properties. Like lavender, it can be dabbed directly on blemishes.

AROMATIC FACIAL BLENDS

Try some of these evocative essential-oil combinations, designed to give your face a real boost.

Eastern serenity: Blend 2 tablespoons carrier oil, 3 drops patchouli essential oil, 2 drops sandalwood essential oil, and 2 drops jasmine essential oil.

English rose: Blend 2 tablespoons carrier oil, 5 drops rose essential oil, 3 drops rose geranium oil, and 2 drops lavender essential oil.

Tropical treat: Blend 2 tablespoons carrier oil, 4 drops mandarin oil, 2 drops neroli, and 2 drops ylang ylang.

Southwestern breeze: Blend 2 tablespoons carrier oil, 4 drops sage oil, 2 drops cedarwood, and 2 drops lavender oil.

SPECIAL RECIPES

Try these essential oil blends for treating specific skin conditions.

Skin hydrator for parched, dry skin: Blend 2 tablespoons of carrier oil with 3 drops of lavender oil, 2 drops of neroli oil, and 2 drops of patchouli oil.

Wake-up treat for fatigued, lackluster skin: Blend 2 tablespoons of carrier oil with 4 drops of sandalwood oil, 3 drops of jasmine oil, and 3 drops of rose oil.

Post-sun reviver for over-exposed skin: Blend 2 tablespoons of carrier oil with 5 drops of chamomile and 5 drops of lavender oil.

Break-out blend for zapping blemishes: Blend 1 tablespoon of carrier oil with 5 drops of bergamot oil, 5 drops of tea tree oil, and 5 drops of lavender oil. Dab on individual blemishes.

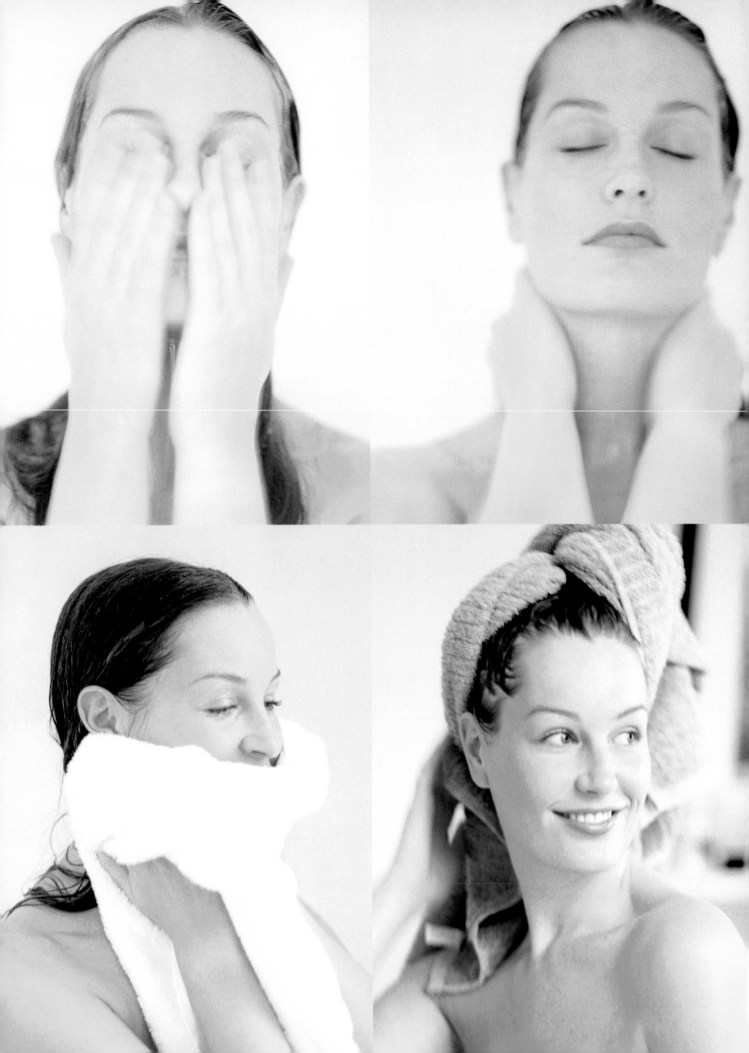

Do-it-yourself facials

Even the dullest complexion will glow after this revitalizing facial routine devised by spa company Li'Tya for Daintree Eco-Lodge and Spa in Australia.

1. Cleanse

1 tsp juice of lime
1 tsp liquid honey
1 tsp lemon myrtle tea infusion (prepare 1 cup of tea, to be used during steaming and exfoliation processes, tea leaves as well as the tea liquor)
2 tbsp natural yogurt
1 tbsp baked yam
1 drop wild lavender essential oil
1 drop mandarin essential oil

Blend all the ingredients in listed order, adding the essential oils last. Add a little more lemon myrtle tea infusion if the mixture is too thick.

2. Steam

4½ cups boiling water
3 leaves lemon myrtle
3 leaves eucalyptus
1 tbsp fresh peppermint leaves or 2 drops peppermint essential oil

In a large bowl, dilute the remaining lemon myrtle tea infusion with the boiling water. Then add the rest of the ingredients to the infusion. Cover your head and the bowl with a large towel to receive maximum benefit from steaming. Remain under the steam for at least 5 minutes.

3. Exfoliate

1 tsp finely grated lime zest
1 tbsp eucalyptus honey
1 tsp ground macadamia nuts

Remove the lemon myrtle, eucalyptus, and fresh peppermint leaves from the steam bowl and chop them finely. If the lemon myrtle tea infusion was made with a tea bag, add the contents to this mixture of leaves. Then add the fresh ingredients listed above.

Gently massage the mixture on your face and throat, taking care around the eye area. To remove, wet a washcloth with warm water and wipe your face. Rinse your face with a cool splash of water to complete this step. Pat dry with a clean towel.

4. Mask

2 tbsp heavy cream
1 tbsp eucalyptus honey
2 tsp dried lavender flowers
2 tsp fresh jasmine flowers
1 tsp grated mandarin zest (optional)

Make a mixture from the ingredients, first whipping together the cream and honey. Add the flowers and mandarin zest, and mix well before applying to your face. Leave the mask on your face for 15 to 20 minutes. To remove, wet a washcloth with warm water and wipe off gently.

5. Hydrate

Complete the facial by applying a small amount of macadamia oil (or a light vegetable or nut oil) and blotting with a tissue.

Eastern facial

Is your skin in need of an overhaul? Try this deluxe facial inspired by recipes from Indonesian spas including The Mandara Spas at The Chedi in Indonesia and The Datai in Malaysia.

For the scrub
1 tbsp dry corn kernels
1 tbsp ground rice powder
1 tbsp cucumber juice for oily skin or 1 tbsp carrot juice for normal/dry skin

For the mask
2 tbsp clay powder
1 tbsp cucumber juice for oily skin or 1 tbsp carrot juice for normal/dry skin

1. For the scrub, mix the corn kernels with the rice powder and add either cucumber or carrot juice depending on your skin type. Massage into damp, freshly cleansed skin.
2. Remove the scrub with warm water and a muslin cloth, massaging gently as you go.
3. Mix the clay and the cucumber or carrot juice to make a mask and use a pastry brush to brush it onto your face, avoiding the eye area.
4. Leave on for 10 to 15 minutes and remove with warm water and a muslin cloth.
5. Pat your skin dry and use a little rose or sandalwood facial oil to moisturize your skin, using your fingertips to tap lightly across your face to stimulate your circulation.

Traditional Thai facial

Simple ingredients yield potent results in this traditional Thai-style facial based on a recipe used for many centuries by Thai women. Variations are available at many Indonesian and Thai spas, including The Banyan Tree Spa in Indonesia and Thailand. If you thought cucumbers were the staple of teenage beauty treatments, think again.

1 cup clear honey
10 drops fresh lime juice
1 medium-sized cucumber, thinly sliced, rind removed

1. Cleanse your face with warm water and a muslin cloth.
2. Mix the honey and lime juice together and pat on to your face, massaging it in thoroughly for 10 to 15 minutes.
3. Remove the honey with warm water and a muslin cloth.
4. Lie down, and place the cucumber slices over your entire face, allowing them to overlap.
5. Leave for 10 minutes while you relax and practice deep breathing.
6. Rinse your skin with cool water and pat dry.
7. Finish by applying a little soy oil to moisturize.

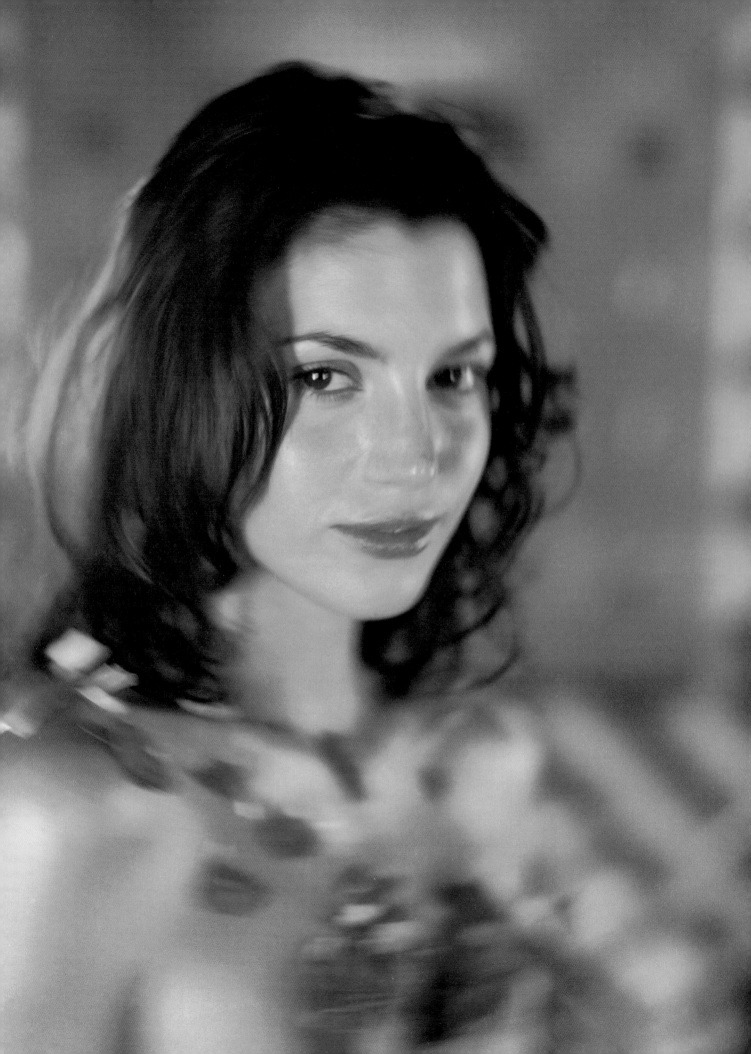

Cleansing and toning

Give your skin-care routine a makeover with freshly made cleansers, masks, and scrubs straight from the recipe books of spas across the globe. They not only prove that treating your skin can be fun rather than a chore, but that beauty doesn't have to cost an arm and a leg.

Yogurt and polenta scrub

Gently slough away dead skin with this super-cleansing facial polish from The Mandara Spa at The Chedi in Indonesia.

2 tbsp natural yogurt
1 tbsp polenta

1. Mix the yogurt and polenta into a paste and gently rub into damp skin with your fingertips.
2. Work your way outward, starting from the center of your forehead to your hairline, down your nose, and along your cheeks to your ears, and from your mouth to your chin and across your jaw line.
3. Rinse away with warm water and a muslin cloth.

Tropical facial scrub

Treat skin to this tropical treat inspired by traditional Asian spa recipes and made with a combination of zingy citrus ingredients and delicious soothing honey and jasmine oil.

3 tbsp ground oatmeal or polenta
1 tsp freshly grated orange peel
1 tsp freshly squeezed lemon or lime juice
1 tsp clear honey
1 tsp coconut oil
2 drops jasmine oil

1. Combine all the ingredients in a blender until you have a smooth paste.
2. Massage into your skin with your fingertips using a circular motion.
3. Rinse with warm water.

Honey and oil cleanser

For a deep-cleaning experience, try this cleanser, inspired by a recipe from The Jamu Traditional Spa in Indonesia.

2 tsp clear honey
3 tsp olive or coconut oil
1 drop frankincense essential oil

1. Blend together the honey, oil, and frankincense essential oil.
2. Apply to your face with your fingertips and massage into your skin.
3. Leave on for 2 to 3 minutes, then rinse off with warm water.
4. Pat your skin dry.

Exotic neroli and patchouli cleanser

Synonymous with Bali, patchouli is renowned for its healing action on the skin, while neroli, a natural sedative, calms and soothes the skin.

1 tbsp sweet almond oil
1 tbsp jojoba oil
3 drops neroli essential oil
3 drops patchouli essential oil
1 oz cocoa butter
½ oz beeswax
1 tbsp orange flower water
¼ tsp borax (available at drugstores)

1. Combine all the oils and cocoa butter in a double boiler. Add the beeswax, a little at a time, and stir in until it melts.
2. Warm the orange flower water in a small pan and stir in the borax.
3. Add to the oil mixture and mix well. Leave to cool and thicken.
4. When cool, put into a dark glass jar. Keep refrigerated and use within four weeks.
5. To use, massage the mixture into your skin to dissolve traces of makeup and grime. Blot and finish off with a spritz of Lemon Refresher (see opposite page for recipe).

Leila's peachy mask

Leila Fazel, co-creator of Agua at Delano in Florida, and Agua at Sanderson in London, shares her all-time favorite facial treat based on a traditional recipe that she learned from her Iranian-born mother.

2 tbsp natural yogurt
2 tbsp peeled and mashed peaches
½ tsp baking soda
1 drop hydrogen peroxide (optional)

1. Make a mixture of the yogurt, peeled and mashed peaches, baking soda, and hydrogen peroxide (if using). Apply the mixture to your face and let it dry while you sip some herbal tea.
2. Once dry, wipe away with a warm washcloth and moisturize with a very thin layer of soy oil.

Aloe and lavender cooler

Based on a facial recipe from The Jimbaran Spa at The Four Seasons Resort in Bali, Indonesia, this mask is ideal for weather-beaten skin.

2 tbsp aloe vera gel
5 drops lavender essential oil

1. Mix the aloe vera gel with the lavender oil.
2. Place in the refrigerator to chill for 20 minutes.
3. Apply to your face, avoiding the eye area, and leave for 15 minutes.
4. Rinse off with tepid water.

Rosy tonic

This fragrant tonic is the perfect English-style toner for dry or mature skins.

½ cup distilled water
8 drops rose essential oil
4 drops glycerine
¼ cup witch hazel

1. Combine all the ingredients in a dark glass bottle and shake well.
2. Transfer to an atomizer and store in the refrigerator for a refreshing spritz.

Aromatic honey toner

Reminiscent of traditional Malaysian skin tonics, this honey water leaves your skin feeling wonderfully refreshed.

¼ tsp clear honey
1 tsp cider vinegar
½ cup distilled water
2 drops neroli essential oil
1 drop ylang ylang essential oil
1 drop sandalwood essential oil

1. Add the honey, vinegar, and 1 tablespoon of the water to a double boiler and heat gently until the honey has dissolved.
2. Pour into a dark glass bottle and add the essential oils and the remaining water.
3. Store in a cool place; it keeps for two weeks.
4. Splash on your skin after applying a mask or scrub. Leave for 30 minutes before rinsing off.

Santa Fe-style spritzer

Based on the sage native to the area surrounding the Ten Thousand Waves' Japanese-style spa, New Mexico, USA, this toner will leave your skin feeling tingly and refreshed.

3 tbsp dried sage
3 tbsp ethyl alcohol
¼ tsp borax
2 tbsp witch hazel
10 drops glycerine
2 drops sage essential oil
2 drops juniper essential oil

1. Place the dried sage and the alcohol in a bowl, cover, and leave for 10 to 14 days. Strain, saving the liquid.
2. In a bowl, dissolve the borax in the witch hazel, and stir in the sage liquid. Add the glycerine and essential oils and pour into a dark glass bottle. Keep in a cool place and shake before use.

Lemon refresher

Based on a traditional Balinese spa recipe, this citrus spritz is the ideal refresher for oily skins.

1 lemon or lime, juiced
2 tbsp distilled water

1. Strain the lemon or lime juice, add to the water, and mix. Place in a plastic atomizer and chill in the refrigerator.
2. Spritz on your skin after applying one of the masks or scrubs included in this chapter.

Face your problems

Sometimes skin demands intensive care or special measures to bring it back into balance. Seasonal changes, hormonal swings, environmental factors, and stress levels can all add up to out-of-control skin. Designed to combat everything from desert-dry skin to an overly oily complexion, here are some favorite spa skin-saving solutions.

Aromatic facial steam

Steam baths and saunas are synonymous with spas. Excellent for cleansing and decongesting, try this aromatic sauna, especially for skin that is unbalanced or is prone to blemishes.

2 drops tea tree essential oil
2 drops lavender essential oil
1 drop sage essential oil
1 sprig fresh rosemary

1. Cleanse your face. Dab a little eye cream around your eyes to protect the skin and apply lip balm to your lips.
2. Fill a large bowl with freshly boiled water and add the essential oils and fresh rosemary.
3. Cover your head with a towel and place your face over the bowl, ensuring that you are not too close to the boiling water.
4. Steam for about 5 minutes.

Lip soother

If your lips feel as dry as the Mojave Desert, try this to-die-for lip balm recipe created by Cindy Fitzgerald at the Golden Door.

3 tsp beeswax
3 tsp almond oil

1. In a small double boiler, melt the beeswax.
2. Add the almond oil and mix well.
3. Pour into a small, thick glass jar and leave to cool.
4. Massage into your lips to rehydrate and soothe.

Instant calmer

Masks are part and parcel of many spa facials, not only because of their effective deep-cleansing action, but because they deliver ingredients to the skin quickly and effectively. Ideal for intensive care, this soothing mask is a boon if your skin is going through a period of unrest or is overly sensitive.

1 tsp green clay
1 tsp oatmeal
1 tsp ground almonds
3 tbsp orange flower water
½ tsp vitamin E oil
1 drop neroli essential oil
1 drop sandalwood essential oil

1. Blend the clay, oatmeal, and almonds with the orange flower water to form a paste.
2. Add the vitamin E and essential oils, and mix well.
3. Smooth on to your face, avoiding the eye area, and leave for 15 minutes.
4. Remove with warm water and a muslin cloth, pressing gently at first to loosen the mask.

Aromatic face saver

This recipe, created by Cindy "Hilani" Woodward from the Golden Door, calms, heals, and comforts dry skin—the very best of face savers.

2 tbsp aloe vera gel
1 vitamin E capsule
½ tsp vanilla extract or 2 drops vanilla essential oil

1. Pre-chill the aloe vera gel in the refrigerator.
2. Break open the vitamin E capsule and combine it with the vanilla extract or oil.
3. Whip all the ingredients together until frothy and apply to your face for 10 to 15 minutes.
4. Remove with warm water and a muslin cloth or washcloth.

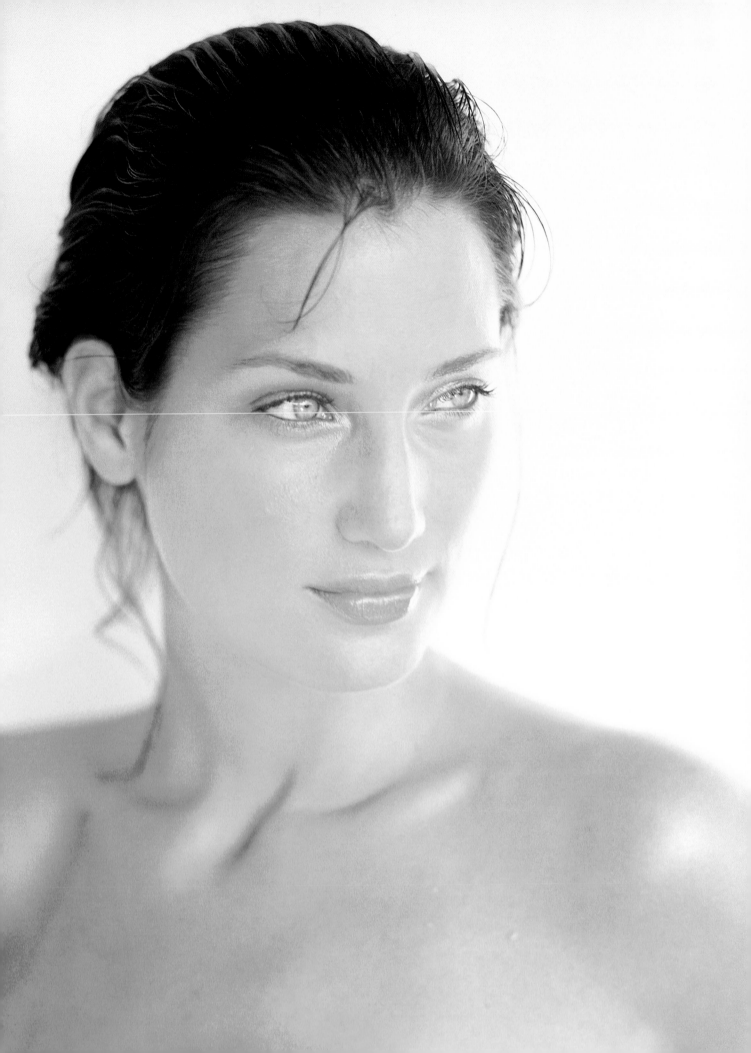

Hands and feet

Often neglected and always taken for granted, hands and feet are often the last to be indulged in pampering treats. Always included on spa menus, take your pick from these revitalizing recipes and regimes.

Pampering pedicure

Created by Suzanne Chavez, spa therapy director at Vista Clara Ranch Resort and Spa in New Mexico, this treatment will ensure the smoothest, sleekest feet.

1 basin or large bowl
1¾ pints warm to hot water
1 capful vinegar or 5 drops lavender essential oil

1. Find a comfortable chair and put on your favorite movie, radio program, or music.
2. Fill your pedicure basin or bowl with the warmest water you can tolerate.
3. Add the vinegar or lavender essential oil.
4. Soak your feet for at least 10 minutes.
5. Use your pedicure file to vigorously remove the rough edges on your feet. Place feet back in tub and soak again while you sit back and relax.
6. Then choose one of the ideas given below.

EXTEND YOUR PEDICURE

To relax: Cover your feet entirely with a facial mask; prop up your feet wrapped in a warm, steamy, damp towel. When through, rinse and apply your favorite lotion.
To invigorate: Combine enough salt and oil to mix easily and massage your feet thoroughly. Then dip your feet once again into the tub to rinse away the salt and pat dry.
To heal: Apply comfrey salve or lavender oil and prop up your feet, relax, and finish that movie!

Hand and wrist massage

Treat hands to this super-moisturizing and relaxing massage. It's ideal for alleviating tension, particularly if you work at a keyboard.

2 tsp sweet almond or jojoba oil
2 drops camomile essential oil
2 drops lavender essential oil

1. Blend all the ingredients together in a small heatproof cup. Place the cup in a bowl of boiling water, ensuring that the water level is about half-way up the cup. Let it stand for about 5 minutes to warm the oil.
2. Warm your hands by rubbing them briskly together or placing them in a bowl of warm water for a few minutes.
3. Pour the oil on your hands and massage it well into your wrists, palms, and fingers, using firm, even pressure. Finish by patting your hands dry with a towel to remove excess oil.

Floral foot soak

Treat tired feet to this restorative footbath, based on the recipe from the spa at The Bali Hyatt.

½ cup of pre-blended foot scrub (see scrub recipe overleaf)
3 drops each of thyme, vetiver, and sage essential oils
bowl of warm water
2 tbsp wheatgerm, coconut, or jojoba essential oil
handful of fresh flowers

1. Scrub feet with the foot scrub, rubbing vigorously to remove callused skin and to stimulate circulation. If you have very hard or rough skin, use a pumice stone with the scrub.
2. Rinse feet under the shower. Pat dry.
3. Massage your feet with the blended thyme, vetiver, and sage essential oils, working your way from the toes up to the ankles.
4. Fill a bowl with warm water and add the wheatgerm, coconut, or jojoba essential oil. Throw in the flowers and place your feet in the bowl. Let them soak for 10 to 15 minutes.

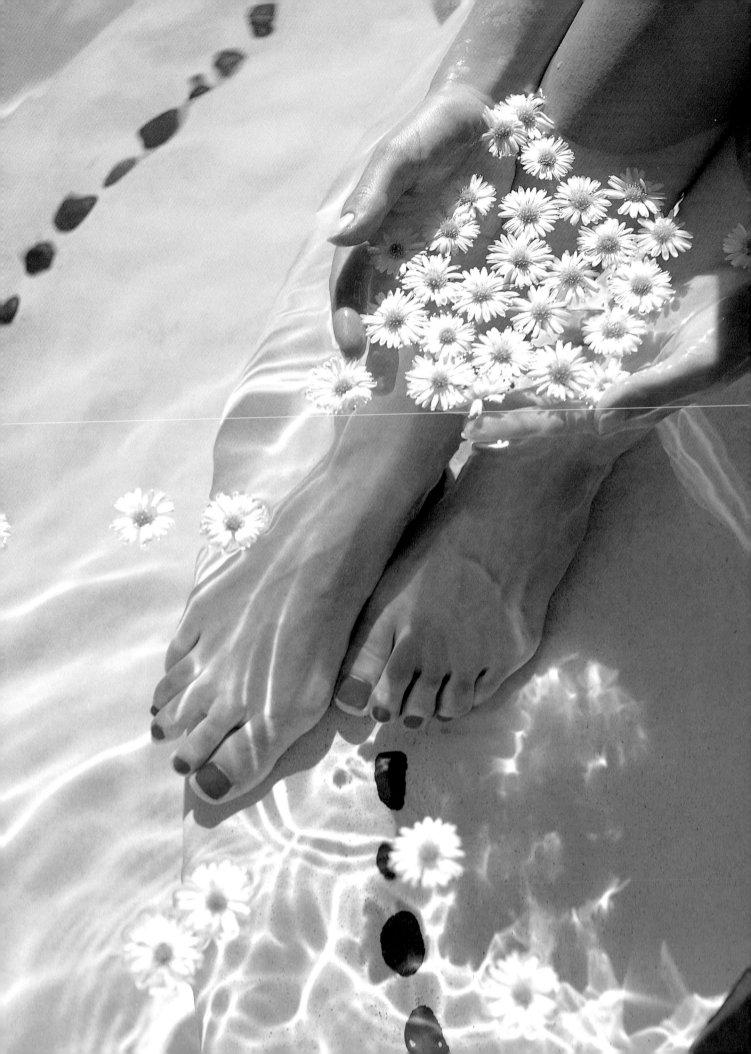

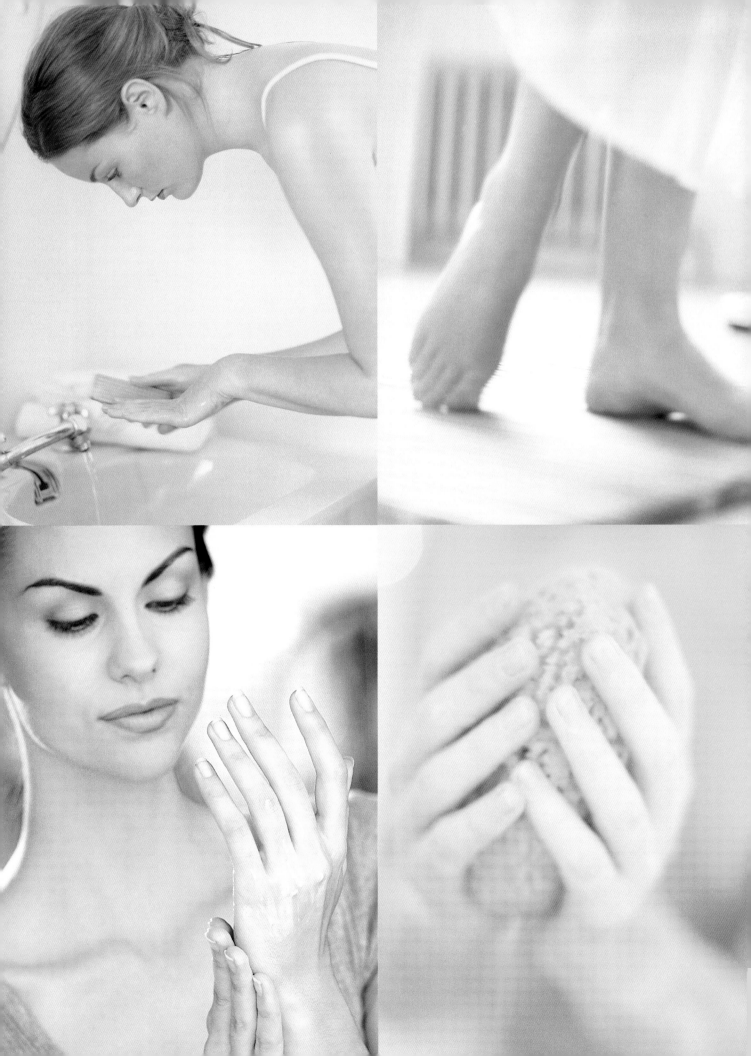

Flower mask for hands and feet

Based on a traditional Balinese spa recipe, this mask will deep cleanse and moisturize both hands and feet.

6 tbsp kaolin or green clay powder
2 tbsp coconut milk
1 tsp ground cloves
1 tsp ground cinnamon
1 tsp ground ginger
handful of rose petals or jasmine flowers
5 drops lavender essential oil

1. Thoroughly combine all the ingredients to make a thick paste.
2. Apply to hands or feet and leave on for 20 minutes or until it dries.
3. Rinse with warm water, gently rubbing to remove traces of the mask.
4. Finish by massaging your hands or feet with coconut or sesame oil.

Nut scrub

Inspired by a recipe at The Jamu Traditional Spa in Bali, this foot scrub will leave feet feeling blissed out and super-smooth.

7 oz lemon grass
2 cups boiling water
1 tbsp almonds
1 tbsp macadamia nuts
1 tsp coconut oil

1. Make an infusion with the lemon grass and boiling water. Let it steep for 20 minutes; then cool and strain; save the liquid in a jug.
2. Blend the nuts, lemon grass infusion, and oil to make a smooth paste.
3. Massage into your feet to help remove dry skin.

Exotic hand cream

For parched hands, try this super-moisturizing recipe, which will leave skin soft and fragrant.

2 tsps honey
¼ cup coconut oil
10 drops pure vitamin E oil
10 drops rose essential oil
10 drops sandalwood essential oil
5 drops ylang ylang essential oil

1. Warm the honey and coconut oil in a double boiler and mix well until combined.
2. Add the vitamin E oil, then the essential oils.
3. Pour into a bowl and allow to cool to a comfortable temperature.
4. Massage into your hands, and allow to soak in for at least 20 minutes before wiping away the excess with a warm, damp washcloth.

All-over body boosters

Whether you are feeling under-the-weather or in need of a general boost, the following spa recipes are designed to zap specific problems, such as colds, aches and pains, fatigued muscles, or problem skin.

Immune booster bath

Inspired by treatments at Israeli spas, such as the Radisson Moriah Plaza Dead Sea Spa Hotel and the Carmel Forest Spa Resort, this bath helps to promote the elimination of acidic wastes from the body by encouraging perspiration. It is particularly excellent if you are suffering from muscular aches and pains and for warding off and treating colds and flu, it's a boon in the winter months.

1 cup Dead Sea salts
4 drops tea tree essential oil
4 drops pine or cedar essential oil
6 drops patchouli oil

1. Add the Dead Sea salts to the bath while it is filling with comfortably hot water. Just before you step in, add the essential oils.
2. Place a few drops of each essential oil into a warm, damp washcloth or piece of muslin and place on your forehead. Soak in the tub for 20 minutes. Wrap up very warmly afterwards and sip a cup of soothing fennel or rosehip tea.

Deep heat boreh scrub

The perfect antidote to a chilly, wintry day or if you are feeling a cold or the flu coming on, this treatment is recommended by The Oberoi in Bali. Recognized as a traditional medicine, it is believed to help warm the body and relieve aching joints, sore muscles, and headaches. It also increases blood circulation. Applied to the skin, it gives a wonderful all-over deep heat sensation. Avoid if you are pregnant, have very sensitive skin, or skin conditions such as eczema.

1 tsp jojoba oil
4 tsp sandalwood powder
2 tsp ginger
2 tsp whole cloves
1 tsp cinnamon
1 tsp coriander seeds
1 tsp nutmeg
1 tsp turmeric
1 tsp black pepper
2 tsp rice powder
3 large carrots, grated finely

1. Mix the oil, herbs and spices, and rice powder to make a thick paste. If you have a sensitive skin, it is best to use a larger amount of rice powder and to reduce the amount of spices in the mix by half.
2. Cover your body with the paste and leave on for 5 to 10 minutes while you feel the warming sensation.
3. Massage it into your skin until it begins to slough off.
4. Follow by rubbing the carrot into your skin to moisturize.
5. Shower off and moisturize with a lotion.

Mandi Kimiri dry skin booster

For post-holiday skin that's paper dry, this intensive body smoother is more than a mere exfoliant. Your skin will feel incredibly soft and moist afterwards. Inspired by a recipe that's exclusive to The Jamu Traditional Spa in Bali, it smells so delicious, you'll want to eat it too.

½ cup macadamia nuts
½ cup peeled natural peanuts
1 tbsp freshly grated ginger
1 tbsp avocado or almond oil

1. Grind the nuts in a food processor, add the ginger and the oil, and process until you get a peanut-butter-style paste.
2. Rub the mixture over damp skin, massaging in a firm, circular motion with the palms of your hands.
3. Rinse with warm water and pat your skin dry.

Tonic body rub

If you're feeling unrested after a night's sleep, try this stimulating body rub, inspired by treatments available at many French and Italian spas and based on aromatic ingredients.

1 tbsp cider vinegar
5 drops lemon balm essential oil
5 drops tangerine essential oil
3 drops patchouli essential oil
3 drops juniper essential oil
2 drops rosemary essential oil
1¼ cups orange flower water

1. Add the ingredients to a dark glass bottle and shake thoroughly to blend.
2. Take a warm shower and towel dry your skin vigorously.
3. While you are still standing in the tub or shower, sprinkle the essential oil tonic liberally on to your hands and apply all over your body, working from your feet upward. Your skin will feel tingly, your mood will uplift, and your energy level will improve.

Therapeutic muscle fatigue bath

During a spa vacation, you may find that you've worked your body harder than ever before. Although this is one of the most enjoyable aspects of going to a spa, particularly if it is fitness oriented like The Ashram or Canyon Ranch, you may find that your body aches and your muscles are fatigued after a day of hiking and cycling. Designed to help soothe away any aches, this therapeutic bath recipe is designed to relax and revitalize. Of course, it's just as useful after a day of gardening, a session at the gym, or a long walk.

3 tbsp Epsom salts
2 drops marjoram essential oil
2 drops lavender essential oil
2 drops chamomile essential oil

1. Run a warm bath and add the Epsom salts. Swirl the water around to allow the salts to dissolve. Slip into the bath and add the essential oils.
2. Inhale the aroma deeply as you soak for about 20 minutes. Ensure that you keep warm after your bath.

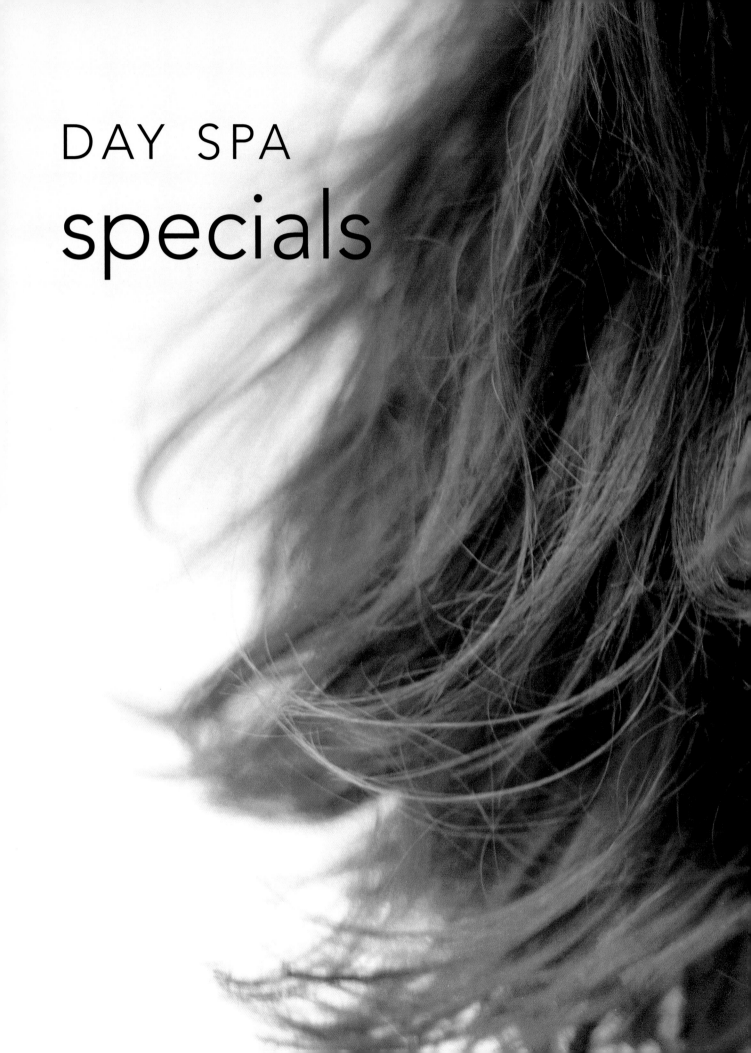

DAY SPA
specials

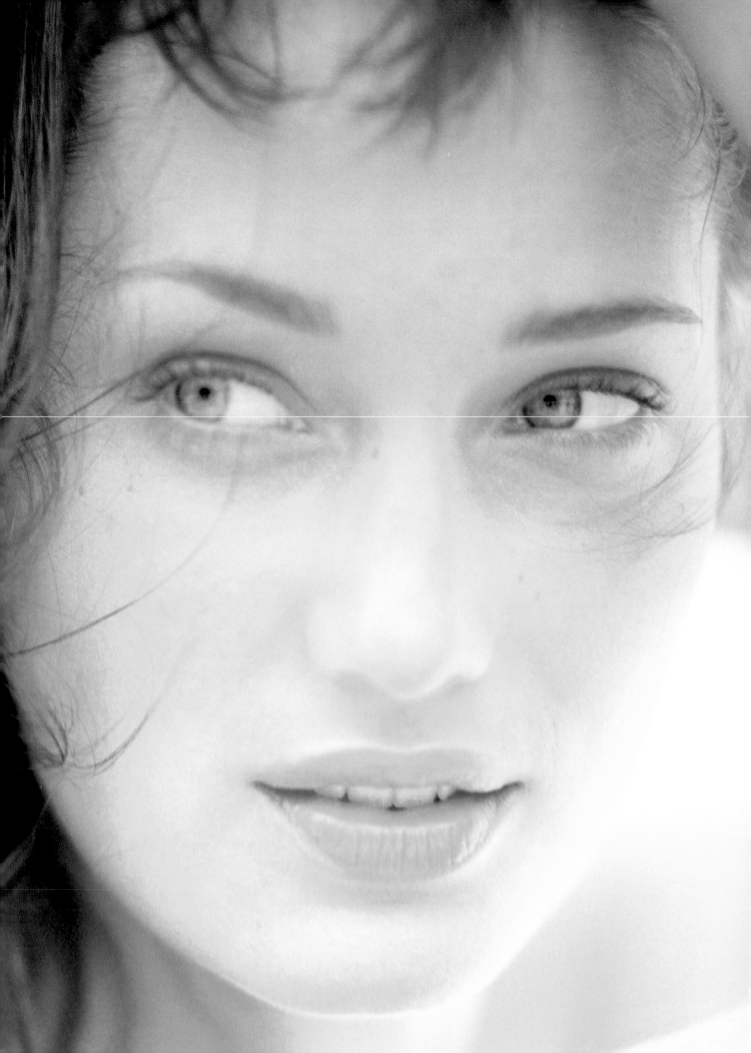

The chill-out day

When stress levels are soaring to an all-time high, dip into this soothing spa-at-home special, with tips and ideas from spas around the world.

DEEP BREATHING

Start your day with some deep breathing. Not only will it increase your energy levels, but it will also help to relax your mind and body.

• Sit on the floor with your legs crossed or on a chair that supports your back with your feet flat on the floor.

• Breathe in slowly, taking the breath through your nose. As you inhale, be conscious of the air passing along your windpipe, into your lungs and diaphragm. Focus on your breath as it travels down.

• Exhale slowly and steadily, ensuring that you are constantly focused on your breathing. Practice this cycle for about 5 minutes.

INSTANT CALMER

Run a warm bath and add to it this soothing bath oil combination from a recipe at the Nusa Dua Spa in Bali.

Tranquility oil: 3 drops of vetiver essential oil, 3 drops of ylang ylang essential oil, and 3 drops of sandalwood essential oil in 2 tablespoons of soy or jojoba carrier oil.

As you soak in the water, try the Desert Healing Breath technique from Westward Look Resort in Arizona, where guests are taught this calming deep-breathing exercise so that they can relax and recall the tranquility of the desert after they return home.

• Close your eyes and picture the colors of the desert sky or a place that you love to visit. Imagine the warm wind blowing against your face, and breathe deeply and slowly in and out to the count of three.

• Absorb the fragrance of this place, hold it briefly, then gently release both your breath and any tension.

• Repeat several times, deepening your relaxation with each exhalation. By focusing on the sights and sounds and stimulations, you can cleanse your mind and spirit.

MEDICINE WALK

Dress in appropriate outdoor clothing and plan a leisurely walk in the park, along the beach, or in a nature reserve near your home. Try this Medicine Walk as experienced by guests at Vista Clara Ranch Resort and Spa in New Mexico. Part of the Spa Ancestral Ways program, it was devised by Julie Rivers and Dona Wilder.

• Nurture yourself by taking a walk with a different point of view.

• In the Native American way, this could be called a Medicine Walk. Walk slowly, feeling your connection to the Earth Mother. Walk in awareness with soft eyes. Allow your eyes to gently scan your surroundings.

• If something catches your attention such as a cloud, a bird, or a stone in your path, take a moment to observe it more closely.

• Listen with soft ears. What is calling you? Is it the wind spirits, the song of the bird, the laughter of children, or the flicker of butterfly wings? What is the message?

• Open your heart as you walk and follow your feelings–hug that tree, skip, dance, or sing– responding to your inner urges. Be fully present in each moment of this walk, as you communicate with All Our Relations.

Calming cucumber and coconut mask

¼ unpeeled cucumber
1 tbsp almond milk (blend 2 tbsp almonds with
½ cup of water in a blender until smooth then
strain through a muslin cloth to extract the milk)
¼ avocado flesh
2 tbsp coconut oil
2 tbsp kaolin powder

1. Blend all the ingredients, apart from the kaolin, in a blender until smooth.
2. Add the kaolin, little by little, to make a paste that is firm but still workable.
3. Apply to your face with a pastry brush or your fingertips and allow to dry for 10 to 15 minutes.
4. Rinse away with warm water. Pat your skin dry.

Complete the calming and relaxing process by giving yourself a head and face massage using a soothing blend of essential oils. Try the Eastern serenity or the Southwestern breeze blends (see page 100).

Soothing herbal tea

Prepare yourself a soothing herbal tea. Try a combination of hops, a natural sedative with valerian, which is tension and anxiety reducing; or blend a little passionflower with orange blossom, both of which will help to induce restful sleep. Prepare an infusion using 1 tbsp of each herb in 1 cup of boiling water. Strain and drink. Sweeten with honey or add a little lemon juice to taste.

10-MINUTE SHIATSU-STYLE MASSAGE

Created by the experts at The Spa at St. David's Hotel, Cardiff, UK, this restorative shiatsu-style massage will not only restore a glow to your face but will work at a deeper level on the rest of the body.

1. Use downward pressure and press three times with the pad of one finger on each hand to stimulate the points in the following way:
Start with the point located in the center of the chin and work your way through each point from 1 to 10 (see diagram) in sequence.

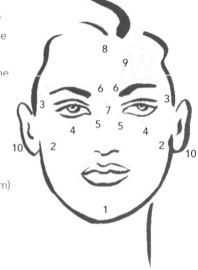

2. Repeat the sequence two or three times.
3. Finish by using light, sweeping finger movements as indicated by the arrow above to stimulate lymphatic drainage. Work toward the temples, ears, and jaw line, as shown in the diagram. This will help to reduce puffiness and dark circles around the eyes.

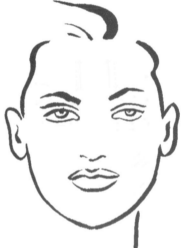

The wake-up call day

Feeling sluggish? In need of a some physical maintenance? Boost your energy level and get your body into gear with this action-packed day. First try these muscle toning exercises recommended by the fitness experts at Lucknam Park, Wiltshire, UK, and then move on to some invigorating massage.

Squats: Stand straight with your feet shoulder-width apart. Bend your knees until your thighs are parallel to the ground. Keep your knees in line with your toes and over the ankles. Return to the starting position and repeat 10 to 15 times.

Lunges: Stand up straight with your feet shoulder-width apart. Take a big step forwards with one leg. Keep the knee just over the ankle and then bend your back leg so that the knee nearly touches the ground. Return the back knee so that it is straight, then bring back your front leg so that you return to a standing position. Repeat 10 to 15 times.

Sit-ups: Lie down with your back flat on the ground. Your knees should be bent and arms out straight above your thighs, and keep your chin up away from your chest. Raise your upper body until your fingertips touch or go past your knees, then return to starting position and do a further 10 to 15 repetitions.

Walk this way: One of the best ways to get fit and to maintain fitness is to powerwalk. Not only does it get you outside and away from your desk, housework, and day-to-day anxieties, but it is incredibly easy to fit into a busy schedule. Plan to take a moderate-to-brisk paced walk of at least 30 minutes duration. (See pages 82–3 for a walking program.)

POST-WORKOUT COOLER

Quench your thirst and refresh your palette with this low-calorie smoothie, a favorite of Leila Fazel, co-founder of Agua at Delano in Florida, and Agua at Sanderson in London. Combine 2 cups frozen honey dew melon, 2 tbsp fresh mint, 1 tbsp lime juice and 1/3 cup ginger ale with six ice cubes in a blender until slushy. Drink, relax, and sit back, contemplating what you have just achieved.

Feet treat

If you've been busy working out, the chances are that your feet will be in need of some attention, no matter how supportive your training shoes are. Try these soothing foot remedies.

1. Massage your feet with sesame or olive oil and a few drops each of tea tree, eucalyptus, and peppermint essential oils. This will help to soothe tired, hot feet and also has the benefit of acting as a natural deodorant.
2. If your feet are very callused, scrub them with a body scrub, rinse with warm water, and cover with cocoa butter. Wrap your feet in plastic wrap and put on a pair of socks. Leave for at least an hour.
3. Give your feet a foot bath by adding a handful of fresh sage, lavender, or bay leaf and a tablespoon of sea salt to a basin of hot water. Soak your feet for at least 10 minutes.

Post-sports massage

When you have been working out, treat your body to a soothing, muscle-relaxing massage.

1 tbsp soy or avocado oil
10 drops marjoram essential oil
4 drops ginger essential oil
3 drops black pepper essential oil

1. Blend all the ingredients together in a dark glass bottle.
2. Pour a little in the palm of your hand to warm it up, then use smooth sweeping movements, working upward and toward the heart, to massage your feet, legs, buttocks, upper arms, shoulders, and stomach.

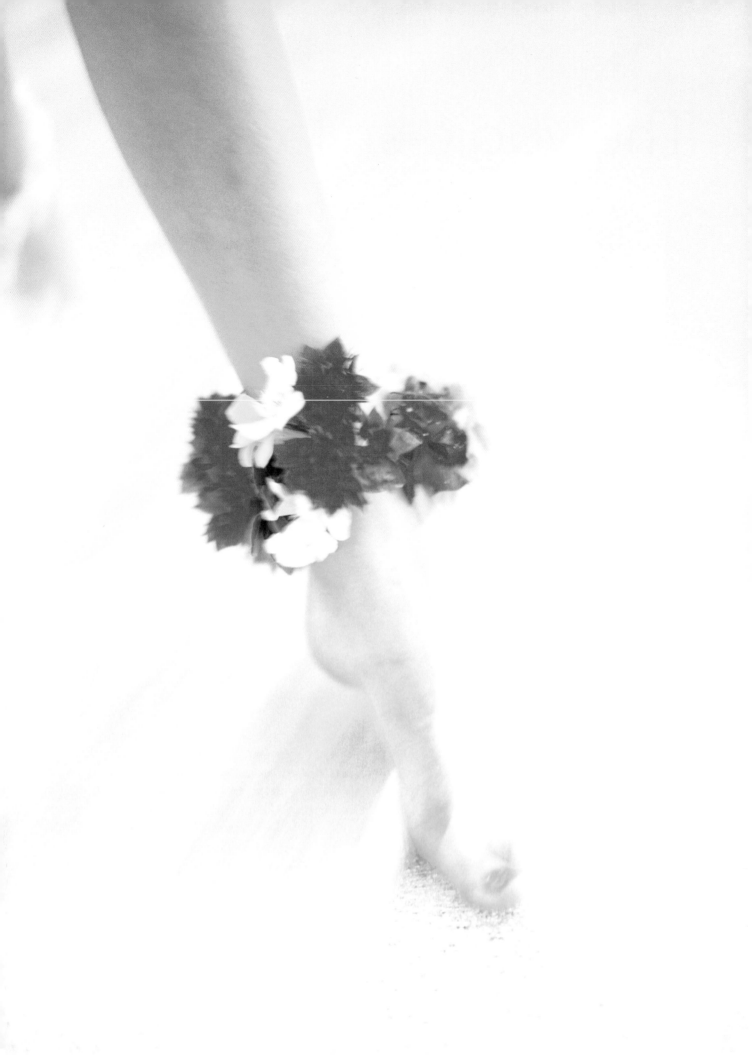

The yogic-style day

Many spas, East and West, now offer a wide range of ayurvedic and yogic therapies as part of their programs. If you are feeling stuck in a rut and in need of a kick-start, try this yogic-style spa day.

THE YOGIC DIET

The yogic way of eating is based on ancient Indian teachings that suggest that all the energy in the universe, including food, has three qualities –inertia or darkness, known as tamas; purity, called sattva; and activity or passion, called rajas. Tamasic foods, including fish, eggs, alcohol, vinegar, and fried and barbecued foods, produce lethargy and a feeling of bloatedness when eaten in excess. Rajasic foods such as garlic, onions, spiced and salted foods, soft drinks and chocolate, and tea and coffee, can upset the balance of mind and body by over-stimulating the mind and making you feel restless and stressed. Sattvic foods, which include milk, butter, cheese, fresh and dried fruits, salads, grains, fresh herbs, nuts, and seeds, are, on the other hand, calming and easy to digest. They also help to boost stamina and intellect. Try to ensure that you steer clear of rajasic and tamasic foods and boost your intake of sattvic foods.

Nourishing coconut rice and vegetables
Makes 2 servings

Try this very simple ayurvedic-style soup, designed to revitalize the mind, body, and soul from The Taj Ayurvedic Center at the Taj Residency in India.

1 cup rice
½ onion, peeled and sliced
1½ carrots, peeled and sliced
1 cup baby corn, sliced
¼ head of broccoli, stalks removed and broken into florets
4 scallions, green parts removed and white parts sliced thinly
⅓ cup coconut milk
salt
1 tsp chopped coriander, to garnish

1. Cook the rice in plenty of boiling salted water for approximately 15 minutes. Drain, retaining about 1½ cups of the cooking water, and set aside the cooked rice.
2. Brown the onion in a non-stick pan.
3. Add and heat the rice water and then add the carrots. Boil for approximately 5 minutes.
4. Add the corn, broccoli, and scallions to the pan with the carrots and the cooked onion, and cook for 5 to 10 minutes longer, until the vegetables are soft.
5. Reduce the heat and stir in the coconut milk. Do not re-heat the soup after adding the coconut milk or it will curdle. Season and serve, garnished with a few spoonfuls of boiled rice and the chopped coriander.

Five-minute yoga sequence

Yoga not only helps to increase flexibility, it also boosts energy levels, relaxes the mind, and improves digestion. Incorporate this yoga sequence, devised by Jennifer Fox and Paul Gould, fitness instructors from Rancho La Puerta, Baja California, Mexico, based on Iyengar yoga.

MOUNTAIN (TADASANA)

Stand evenly balanced on your feet. Pull up through your thighs. Maintaining the natural curves of your spine, try to stand as straight as possible. Imagine that you are a soaring mountain, centered and rising up strongly.

CHAIR (UTKATASANA)

Stretch your arms straight up, lower your thighs toward a parallel line with the ground. Keep your chest as far back as possible and breathe naturally through your nose. You are transforming rounded and stiff shoulders as you fully expand the chest for better posture and deeper breathing.

UPWARD DOG (URDHVAH MUKHA SVANASANA)

Pressing your palms into a low ledge or bench, bring your pelvis and base of spine forward and lightly contract your buttocks. Work your legs back without bending or resting your knees. Keep your chest lifted and shoulders rolled back. In this movement you are opening the upper chest, strengthening the backs of your arms.

DOWNWARD DOG (ADHO MUKHA SVANASANA)

Straighten your legs, lift your hips, and pull back your thighs for an invigorating stretch of the legs, shoulders, and arms. Stay in the posture for 15 seconds to 1 minute and breathe deeply. Repeat twice. The dog pose helps to reduce fatigue and boost energy.

Traditional Indian-style milk bath

Based on ancient Indian milk bath recipes, this particular one will leave your skin smooth and your mind relaxed.

1 cup fresh milk
1 tsp oatmeal
2 drops rose essential oil

1. Mix the milk, oatmeal, and rose essential oil together, then pour into a warm bath.
2. Relax in the bath for at least half an hour.

Traditional Indian-style body polish

This skin-buffing recipe is handed down from generation to generation by Indian women.

2 tbsp fresh milk
1 tbsp chick pea flour
pinch turmeric

1. Mix together all the ingredients.
2. Massage into damp skin to cleanse, buff, and moisturize.

The aqua-therapy day

Water has long been associated with well-being and for many of us, an invigorating shower or relaxing bath is all the therapy we need when we are stressed out or feeling below par. Indulge in a day of water therapy to recharge your batteries and reduce stress levels.

HEALING HOT WATER

Ditch all caffeinated beverages, such as coffee and soda, and exchange them for water or herbal tisanes. For indigestion, try peppermint; for anxiety, headaches, and water retention, try chamomile; for colds and flu, try cinnamon or nutmeg, and to boost your mood, sip lemon balm.

DIP IN

One of the most therapeutic ways to keep fit, swimming not only tones muscles and increases aerobic fitness, but it is also incredibly relaxing. Aim to spend at least an hour in the pool, using a combination of different strokes to work on different parts of your body.
• Backstroke: good for shoulders and promoting relaxation.
• Breaststroke: excellent for toning upper arms and inner thighs.
• Butterfly: the best stroke for building stamina and for aerobic endurance.
• Crawl: a great aerobic workout, this stroke also tones the arms and works on the shoulders and upper back muscles.

WATER-TREADING

Many spas, particularly those in Austria, France, and Germany, offer this hydrotherapy treatment as a cure for insomnia, and nervous tension, and to promote general well being. Fill your tub to mid-calf depth with cold water and add a few trays of ice cubes. Wrap your upper body in a warm, terry cloth robe and step into the bath. March on the spot so that one foot comes fully out of the water while the other stays submerged. Stay in for 1 minute initially and build up gradually until you are treading water for about 3 minutes. Afterwards, dry your feet and legs thoroughly, wrap up warmly, and put on some thick socks to sustain that feeling of relaxation.

Cleopatra dreamsicle bath

For a rejuvenating bathing experience, try this exotic recipe from Cindy "Hilani" Woodward at the Golden Door—it is guaranteed to turn your bath into Nirvana.

½ cup milk
1 sliced orange

1. Add the milk to a warm bath under a running tap.
2. Wrap the sliced orange in a muslin cloth and squeeze into the water to release the oil and juice.
3. Lie back and enjoy the heavenly aroma.

Eye bath

Refresh tired, computer-strained eyes with a soothing eye bath made with water and herbs.

2 cups water
2 tsp dried eyebright or agrimony

1. Add the herbs to the water and boil for 20 minutes.
2. Strain and allow to cool, then pour into two egg cups and use to bathe each eye separately.
3. Soak two cotton pads in the water and use as compresses on your eyes.

Skin booster

While drinking at least eight glasses of water a day is the best way to ensure that skin hydration levels are maintained, this facial hydrotherapy treatment will tone and tighten skin. Use a hand-held shower and cool water to wash your face with a steady flow of water. Hold your head forward over the bath and hold the shower as close to your face as is comfortable. Circle the shower around your face in a clockwise direction and repeat this three to five times before spraying counter-clockwise. Next, concentrate the spray on your forehead for 30 seconds, your temples, and then your jawline. Pat your skin dry.

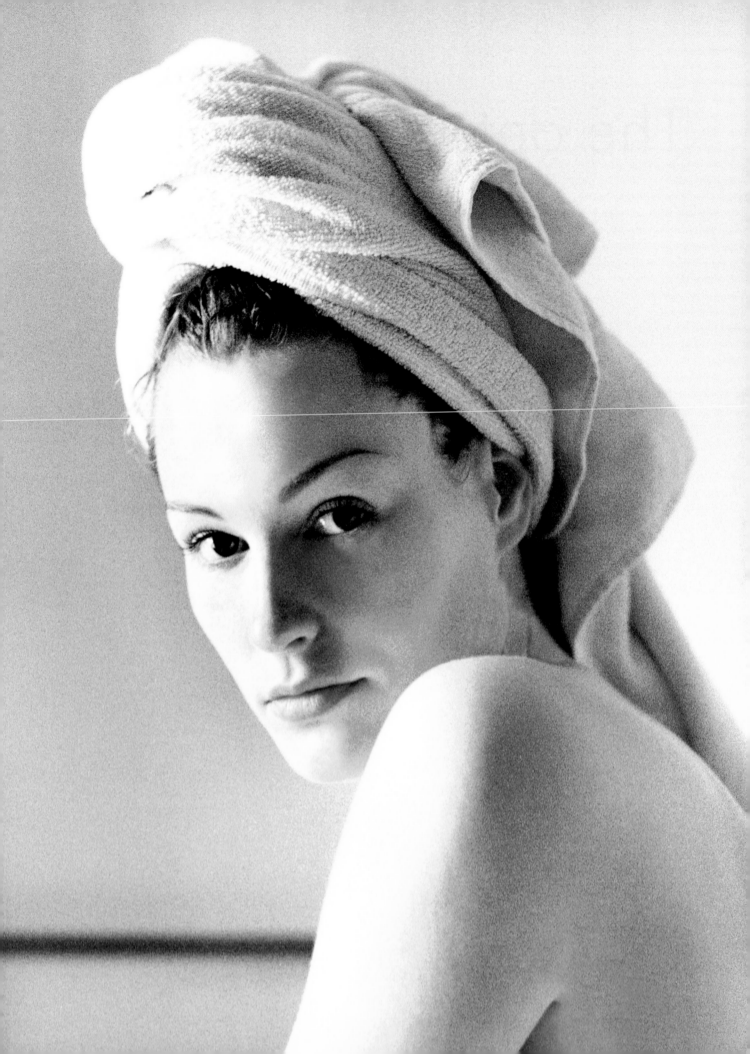

The detox day

If your energy levels are low, your skin and hair looking less than lustrous, and you have been over-indulging of late, try a few of these cleansing treats for the perfect detox day.

DETOX DRINKS

Start the day with a cleansing drink. Squeeze the juice of half a lemon into a cup of freshly boiled water or into freshly squeezed orange juice and sip. Alternatively, brew up some peppermint, elderflower, yarrow, or wild thyme tea, all of which will help your body dispose of toxins, such as alcohol.

CLEANSING FOODS

If you are following a detox program, even if it's just for the day, look to the following points:
• Cut down on red meat, refined sugar, pasta, bread and rice, alcohol, coffee and caffeinated beverages such as soda, crackers, cookies, and pre-packaged and convenience foods.
• Instead, stockpile low-toxin foods such as corn, salmon, brown rice, sardines, and organic chicken and turkey.
• Increase your intake of fresh fruits such as apricots, blueberries, raspberries, oranges, apples, and papaya and cleansing vegetables including tomatoes, broccoli, Brussels sprouts, spinach, beets, and celery.
• Drink at least 4 cups of filtered or bottled water while you are detoxing.
• Take 1000 mg of antioxidant-rich vitamin C to help cleanse and revitalize your system.

Clearing your head

If your hair and scalp are in need of some deep cleansing and detoxing, try this intensive treatment, based on a recipe from The Spa at The Bali Hyatt.

1 tbsp macadamia or coconut oil
10 drops eucalyptus, rosemary, cedarwood, or tea tree essential oils
1 mashed avocado
2 tbsp cider vinegar

1. Warm the macadamia or coconut oil in a double boiler or oil burner and add the essential oil of your choice.
2. Apply the warm oil to the roots of your hair and massage down the hair shaft, working toward the ends. Spend a few minutes massaging your scalp with firm, circular movements of your fingertips. Work from the nape of your neck to your crown and then to your forehead.
3. Once your hair is covered with the oil, apply the mashed avocado, concentrating on the ends rather than the scalp.
4. Wrap your head in a hot towel or wear a plastic shower cap.
5. Leave on for 10 to 15 minutes, and then rinse thoroughly with warm water. Shampoo once or twice, rinse again, then pour on the cider vinegar as a final rinse.

Thai mud wrap

Body wraps are renowned for their detoxifying abilities, drawing impurities out of the skin. Try this recipe based on a secret mud mix from The Oriental Spa in Bangkok.

½ cup green clay or kaolin
½ cup organic milk
½ cup sesame oil
½ tsp turmeric powder
½ tsp sandalwood powder

1. Blend the ingredients until a paste is formed.
2. Slather on to your body and wrap yourself in a plastic sheet (a foil survival sheet from camping-supply stores is ideal) and then in several large, warm bath towels.
3. Keep warm for 20 minutes, then unwrap yourself and shower, rinsing the mask away with warm water.

Salty solution

Try this traditional old-style spa salt bath for a deep-cleansing experience. Run a warm bath and add 1½ cups of Epsom salts, 4 drops of sage, and 2 drops of tea tree essential oils. Lie back, head on a rolled-up towel and soak your body, ensuring the water level comes right up to your neck. Keep the water as hot as is comfortable and relax for about 25 minutes. Then slip into bed and ensure you keep your body warm with pyjamas, socks, and a hot-water bottle. Drink lots of water, as your body will lose fluid through perspiration.

Juice it

If you are planning a detox day, incorporate plenty of fresh vegetable and fruit juices into your program. Not only are they excellent sources of vitamins, minerals, and fiber, they are also brilliant detoxifiers. To get the full benefits of fresh juices, you need to drink them as soon as they are blended. You can stick to separate vegetable or fruit combinations or blend fruits and vegetables to increase their therapeutic benefits. Try these combinations:

Fruits: Grapefruit, orange, and lemon; apple and cranberry; orange, papaya, and melon.
Vegetables: Celery, carrot, and beet; tomato and celery; celery, lettuce, and spinach.
Mixed fruit and vegetables: Apple, celery, and fresh root ginger; carrot and pear; carrot, orange, apple, and lemon; beetroot and carrot.

Salt and soy oil scrub

Stimulate your circulation and slough away dead skin cells with an salt and soy oil body scrub.

1 cup sea salt
½ cup soy oil
3 drops sage or eucalyptus essential oil

1. In a bowl, blend all the ingredients roughly.
2. Dampen your skin under the shower. Then grab a handful of the salt and oil mixture and massage into your skin, working from your ankles upwards.
3. Finish with a short spritz of cold water, then back to warm water to rinse the body scrub away.

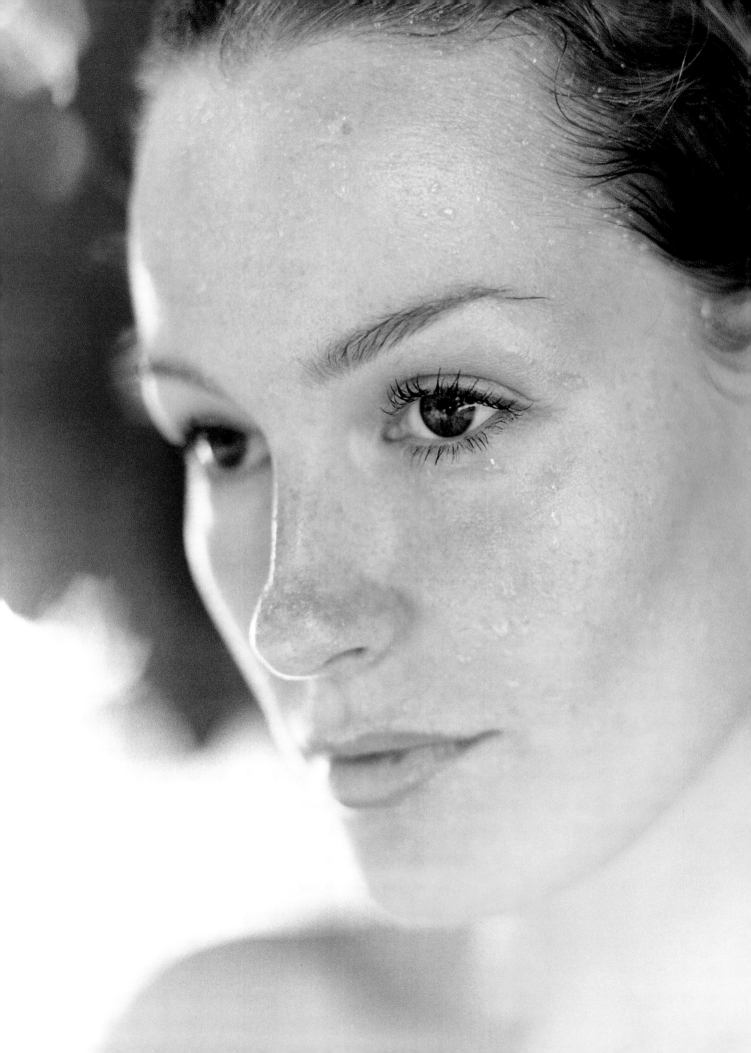

Spa directory

AUSTRALIA

Azabu
End of Skinners Shoot Road
Byron Bay
NSW 2481
Tel: +61 2 6680 9102
Fax: + 61 2 6680 9103
Website: www.azabu.com.au

The Cape Retreat
P.O. Box 810
Byron Bay
New South Wales 2481
Tel: +61 2 6684 1363
Fax: +61 2 6684 3461

Couran Cove Resort Spa and Total Living Centre
P.O. Box 224
Runaway Bay
Queensland 4216
Tel: +61 7 5597 9000
Fax: +61 2 5597 9090

Daintree Eco-Lodge and Spa
20 Daintree Road
Daintree
Queensland 4873
Tel: +61 7 4098 6100
Fax: +61 7 4098 6200

Eaglereach Wilderness Resort
Summer Hill Road
Vacy NSW 2421
Tel: +61 2 4938 8233
Fax: +61 2 4938 8234
Website: www.eaglereach.com.au

Empire Retreat
Caves Road
Yallingup
Western Australia 6282
Tel: +61 8 9755 2065
Fax: +61 8 9755 2297
Website: www.empireretreat.com.au

The Golden Door Health Retreat
Ruffles Road
Willow Vale
Queensland 4209
Tel: +61 7 5546 6855
Fax: +61 7 5546 6173
Website: www.goldendoor.com.au

Hyatt Regency-Coolum
P.O. Box 78
Coolum Beach
Queensland 4573
Tel: +61 7 5446 1234
Fax: +61 7 5446 2957
Website: www.hyatt.com

The Observatory Hotel Spa
89-113 Kent Street
Sydney 2000
Tel: +61 2 9256 2229
Fax: +61 2 9256 2235
Website: www.observatoryhotel.com.au

The Sanctuary Holistic Retreat
P.O. Box 270
Bangalow
New South Wales 2479
Tel: +61 2 6687 1216
Fax : +61 2 6687 1310
Website: www.sanctuary.org.au

Shizuka Ryokan
8 Lakeside Drive
Hepburn Springs
Victoria 3461
Tel: +61 3 5348 2030
Fax: +61 3 5348 1358
Website : www.shizuka.com.au

Solar Springs Health Retreat
96 Osborn Avenue
Bundanoon
New South Wales 2578
Tel: +61 2 4883 6027
Fax: +61 2 4862 1809
Website: www.solar.com.au

AUSTRIA

Hotel Rogner-Bad Blumau
A-8283
Blumau 100
Tel: +43 3383 51000
Fax: +43 3383 5100808
Website: www.rogner.com

CANADA

Banff Springs Hotel and Solace Spa
405 Spray Avenue
Banff
Alberta TOL OCO
Tel: +800-441-1414
Website: www.banffsprings.com

Chateau Lake Louise
111 Lake Louise Drive
Lake Louise
Alberta TOL 1EO
Tel: 403-522-3511
Fax: 403-522-3834
Website: www.cphotels.com

Chateau Whistler
Whistler
British Columbia
Tel: 604-938-2010
Fax: 604-938-2099
Website: www.chateauwhistlerresort.com

Echo Valley Ranch Resort
P.O. Box 16
Clinton
British Columbia BOK 1KO
Tel: 250-459-2386

Hills Health Ranch
P.O. Box 26
108 Mile Ranch
British Columbia VOK 2ZO
Tel: 250-791-5225
Fax: 250-791-6384
Website: www.hillshealthranch.com

Mountain Trek Fitness Retreat and Health Spa
Ainsworth Hot Springs
British Columbia V0G 1AO
Tel: 250-229-5636
Fax: 250-229-5246
Website: www.hiking.com

THE CARIBBEAN

Four Seasons Resort
Box 565
Charlestown
St. Kitts and Nevis
Tel: 869-469-111
Fax: 869-469-1112

Half Moon Club
Halfmoon P.O.
Rose Hall
Montego Bay
Jamaica
Tel: 876-953-2211
Fax: 876-953-2731

La Casa de Vida Natural
P.O. Box 916
Rio Grande
Puerto Rico
Tel: 787-887-4359

La Source
P.O. Box 852
St. Georges
Grenada
Tel: 473-444-2556
Website: www.lasource.com.gd

Le Sport
Cariblue Beach
P.O. Box 437
St Lucia
Tel: 758-450-8551
Fax: 758-450-0368

FRANCE

Caudalie Institut de Vinotherapie
Les Sources de Caudalie
Chemin de Smith Haut-Lafitte
33650 Martillac
Tel: +33 5 57 83 82 82
Fax: +33 5 57 83 82 81

Domaine du Royal Club Evian
Hotel Royal
Rive Suid de Lac de Geneva
74500 Evian-Les-Bains
Tel: +33 4 50 26 85 00

Four Seasons George V
31 Avenue George V
75008 Paris
Tel: +33 01 4952 7000
Fax: +33 01 4952 7010
Website: www.fourseasons.com

Hôtel Ritz
15 Place Vendôme
75001 Paris
Tel: +33 01 4316 3030
Fax: +33 01 4316 3179
Website: www.ritzparis.com

Institute of Thalassotherapy Louison Bobet
Hotel Miramar
13 Rue Louison Bobet
64200 Biarritz
Tel: + 33 5 59 41 30 00

Les Près d'Eugénie-les-Bains
40320 Eugénie-les-Bains
Landes
Tel: +33 05 58 05 0607
Fax: +33 05 58 51 1010

Sofitel Talassa
P.O. Box 10802
56178
Quiberon
Tel: +33 02 9750 2000
Fax: +33 02 9730 4522

GERMANY

Brenner's Park Hotel
Sehiller Strasse 4-6
76530 Baden-Baden
Tel: +49 72 21 9000
Website: www.brenners-park.de

HONG KONG

Mandarin Oriental
5 Connaught Road
Central, Hong Kong
Tel: +85 2 2522 0111
Fax: +85 2 2810 6190

Website: www.mandarin-oriental.com/hongkong

INDIA

The Kairali Ayurvedic Health Resort
Palakkad
Kodumbu
Palakkad District 678551
Kerala
Tel: +91 492 322553
Fax :+91 492 322732
Website: www.kairali.com

The Spa at Rajvilas
Rajvilas Hotel
Goner Road
Jaipur 303 012
Tel: +91 141 640101
Fax: +91 141 640202

The Taj Ayurvedic Centre
Taj Residency
Calicut
Kerala
Tel: +91 492 239939

INDONESIA

Amandari
P.O. Box 33
Kedewatan
Ubud
Bali
Tel: +62 361 975333
Fax: +62 361 975335
Website:
www.amanresorts.com/dari_m.html

The Banyan Tree
Bintan Island
Site A4
Lagoi
Bintan Island
Tel: +62 763 24374
Fax: +62 771 81348
www.banyantree.com/bintan/bintan.htm

Jamu Traditional Spa
KulKulBali
P.O. Box 3097
Denpasar
80030 Bali
Tel: +62 361 752520
Fax: +62 361 752519

The Jimbaran Spa at The Four Seasons Resort
Jimbaran
Denpasar 80361
Bali
Tel: +62 361 701010
Fax: +62 361 701020

The Mandara Spa at The Chedi
Desa Melinggih Kelod Payangan
Gianyar
Ubud ·
Bali 80572
Tel: +62 361 975963
Fax: +62 361 975968
Website: www.mandaraspa.com

The Mandara Spa at The Ibah
Tjampuhan
Ubud
Bali
Tel: +62 361 974466
Fax: +62 361 974467

Nusa Dua Beach Hotel and Spa
P.O. Box 1028
Denpasar
Bali
Tel: +62 361 771210
Fax: +62 361 772621

The Oberoi, Bali
Legian Beach
Jalan Kayu Aya
P.O. Box 3351
Denpasar 80001
Bali
Tel: +62 361 70361
Fax : +62 361 730791
Website: http://www.oberoihotels.com

The Oberoi, Lombok
Medana Beach Tanjung
Mataram 83001 NTB
Lombok
Tel: +62 370 638444
Fax: +62 370 632496

Ritz Carlton
Jalan Karang Mas Sejahtera
Jimbaran
Bali 80364
Tel: +62 361 702222

Spa at The Bali Hyatt
P.O. Box 392
Sanur
Bali
Tel: +62 361 281234
Fax: +62 361 287693
Website: www.hyatt.com

ISRAEL

Carmel Forest Spa Resort
P.O.B. 90000
Haifa 31900
Tel: +972 4 830 7888
Fax: +972 4 832 3988
Website: www.isrotel.co.il

Radisson Moriah Plaza Dead Sea Spa Hotel
Neve Zohar
Dead Sea 86910
Tel: +972 7 659 1591
Fax: +972 7 658 4238

ITALY

Hotel Terme di Saturnia
58050 Saturnia
Tel: +39 05 64 60 1060
Fax: +39 05 64 60 1266

Monsummano Terme Grotta Giusti
Via Grotta 1411
Monsummano Terme
51015
Tel: +39 05 725 1165 or +39 05 725 1008
Fax: +39 05 725 1269
Website: www.grottagiustispa.com

Palazzo Arzaga Spa
25080 Carzago di Calvagese della Riviera
Brescia
Tel: +39 030 68 06 00
Fax: +39 030 68 06 168

MALAYSIA

The Mandara Spa at The Datai
Jalan Telek Datai
07000 Palau Langkawi
Kedah Darul Aman
Tel: +60 4 9592500
Fax: +60 4 9592600

MEXICO

Hosteria Las Quintas
Boulevard Diaz Ordaz 9
Cuernavaca
Morelos CP622 440
Tel: +52 7318 3949

Las Ventanas Al Paradiso
KM 195 Carretera Transpeninsular
San Jose del Cabo
Baja California Sur 23400
Tel: +52 114 40300
Fax: +52 114 40301
Website: www.lasventanas.com

Punta Serena
Km. 20 Carretera Federal 200
Tenacatita-Municipio de la Huerta
48989 Jalisco
Tel: +52 335 15020/15100
Fax: +52 333 515050

Rancho La Puerta
Tecate
Baja California
Tel: +1 760 744 4222
Website: www.rancholapuerta.com

The Spa at Las Ventanas al Paradiso
KM 19.5 Carretera Transpeninsular
San Jose de Cabo
Baja California Sur 23400
Tel: +52 114 40300
Fax: +52 114 40301

MONTE CARLO

Les Thermes Marins de Monte Carlo
Construction begins December 2000
Tel: +37 7 9216 4040
Website: www.montecarloresorts.com

SWEDEN

Spa Selma Lagerlof
Box 500
Sundsberget
68628 Sunne
Tel: +46 565 16610
Website: www.selmaspa.se

SWITZERLAND

Clinique La Prairie
Chemin de la Prairie 2
1815 Clarens
Tel: +41 2 1989 3311
Fax: +41 2 1989 3433
Website: www.laprairie.ch

The Grand Hotel and Spa Victoria-Jungfrau
Hoeheweg 41
3800 Interlaken
Tel: +41 3 3828 2828
Website: www.victoria-jungfrau.ch

Hôtel Les Sources des Alpes
Hoeheweg 41
3954 Leukerbad
Tel: +41 2 7472 2000
Fax: +41 2 7472 2001

THAILAND

The Banyan Tree
33 Moo 4
Srisoonthorn Road
Cherngtalay
Amphur Talang
Phuket 83110
Tel: +66 76 324374
Fax: +66 76 324375

Chiva-Som International Health Resort
73/4 Petchkasem Road
Hua Hin 77110
Tel: +66 32 536536
Fax: +66 32 511154

The Oriental Spa at The Oriental Bangkok
48 Oriental Avenue
Bangkok 10500
Tel: +66 22 360400/ 66 24 397613
Fax: +66 24 397587

UNITED KINGDOM

Agua at Sanderson
50 Berners Street
London W1P 3AD
Tel: +44 (0)20 7300 1414
Fax: +44 (0)20 7300 1415

Apotheke 2020
296 Chiswick High Road
London W4
Tel: +44 (0)20 8995 2293

The Berkeley Health Club and Spa
The Berkeley
Wilton Place
London SW1
Tel: +44 (0)20 7235 6000

Champneys at Tring
Wiggington
Tring
Hertfordshire HP23 6HY
Tel: +44 (0)1441 863351
Fax: +44 (0)1442 872342

Chewton Glen
Christchurch Road
New Milton
Hampshire
Tel: +44 (0)1425 277674

The Cowshed at Babington House
Babington
Nr Frome
Somerset BA11 3RW
Tel: +44 (0)1373 813860

The Dorchester Spa
The Dorchester
55 Park Lane
London W1
Tel: +44 (0)20 7495 7335

Elizabeth Arden Beauty Spa
29 Davies Street
London W1
Tel: +44 (0)20 7629 4488

Forest Mere Health Farm
Liphook
Hampshire
GU30 7JQ
Tel: +44 (0)1428 726000
Fax: +44 (0)1428 723501
Website: www.forestmere.co.uk

Henlow Grange Health Farm
Henlow
Bedfordshire SG16 6DB
Tel: +44 (0)1462 811 111
Fax: +44 (0)1462 815 310
Website: www.henlowgrange.co.uk

Hoar Cross Hall
Hoar Cross
Near Yoxall
Staffordshire DE13 8QS
Tel: +44 (0)1283 575671
Websites:www.hoarcross.co.uk or www.europeanayurveda.com

Le Petit Spa
Malmaison
Piccadilly
Manchester
Tel: +44 (0)161 278 1010

Lucknam Park
Colerne
Nr Bath
Wiltshire
SN14 8AZ
Tel: +44 (0)1225 742777
Website: www.lucknampark.co.uk

Mandarin Oriental
66 Knightsbridge
London SW1
Tel: +44 (0)20 7235 2000

Matt Roberts Urban Spa
One Aldwych
The Aldwych
London WC2
Tel: +44 (0)20 7937 7722

Phillimore Club
45 Phillimore Walk
London W8
Tel: +44 (0)20 7937 2882

Ragdale Hall Health Hydro
Ragdale Village
Nr Melton Mowbray
Leicestershire LE14 3PB
Tel: +44 (0)1664 434831
Fax: +44 (0)1664 434587

The Sanctuary
11 Floral Street
London WC2
Tel: +44 (0)20 7420 5104

St David's Hotel and Spa
Havannah Street
Cardiff Bay
Cardiff CF10 5SD
Tel: +44 (0)2920 313084
Fax: +44 (0)2920 487056
Website: www.rfhotels.com

SPAce NK
127 Westbourne Grove
London W2
Tel: +44 (0)20 7727 8002

Stobo Castle Health Spa
Stobo
Peeblesshire
Scotland EH45 8NY
Tel: +44 (0)1721 760249
Fax: +44 (0)1721 760294

Turnberry Hotel
Turnberry
Ayrshire
Scotland
Tel: +44 (0)1655 331000

UNITED STATES OF AMERICA

ARIZONA

The Boulders Resort
P.O. Box 2090
Carefree, AZ 85377
Tel: 1-888-472-6229 or 480-488-9009
Fax: 480-488-4118

Canyon Ranch Health Resort
8600 East Rockcliff Road
Tucson, AZ 85750
Tel: 520-749-9000
Fax: 520-749-1646
Website: www.canyonranch.com

Center for Well Being at the Phoenician
6000 East Camelback Road
Scottsdale, AZ 85251
Tel: 480-423-2452

Miraval Life in Balance
5000 E. Via Estancia Miraval
Catalina, AZ 85739
Tel: 1-800-825-4000
Website: www.miravalresort.com

The Spa at Marriott's Camelback Inn
5402 East Lincoln Drive
Scottsdale, AZ 85253
Tel: 1-800-24-CAMEL

Westward Look Resort
245 East Ina Road
Tucson, AZ 85704
Tel: 520-297-1151
Fax: 520-297-9023
Website: www.westwardlook.com

CALIFORNIA

The Ashram
2025 North McKain Street
Calabasas, CA 91372
Tel: 818-222-6900
Website: www.theashram.com

Cal-A-Vie
2249 Somerset Road
Vista, CA 92084
Tel: 760-945-2055
Fax: 760-630-0074

Chopra Center for Well Being
7630 Fay Avenue
La Jolla, CA 92037
Tel: 1-888-424-6772 or 858-551-7788
Fax: 858-551-7811

The Expanding Light
14618 Tyler Foote Road
Nevada City, CA 95959
Tel: 1-800-346-5350 or 530-478-7518
Website: www.expandinglight.org

Givency Hotel and Spa
4200 E. Palm Canyon Drive
Palm Springs, CA
Tel: 1-800-276-5000 or 619-770-5000

Golden Door
P.O. Box 463077
Escondido, CA 92046
Tel: 760-744-6677
Fax: 760-591-3048

La Costa Resort & Spa
Costa Del Mar Road
Carlsbad, CA 92009
Tel: 1-800-854-5000 or 760-438-9111
Website: www.lacosta.com

The Lodge at Skylonda
16350 Skyline Blvd.
Woodside, CA 94062
Tel: 650-851-6625
Fax: 650-851-5504

Meadowood
900 Meadowood Lane
St. Helena, CA 94574
Tel: 1-800-458-8080 or 707-963-3646
Fax: 707-963-5863
Website: www.meadowood.com

The Oaks at Ojai
122 E. Ojai Avenue
Ojai, CA 93023
Tel: 1-800-753-OAKS
Website: www.oaksspa.com

Ojai Valley Inn & Spa
Country Club Road
Ojai, CA 93023
Tel: 1-800-422-6524, 1-888-SPA-OJAI or 805-646-1111
Website: www.spaojai.com

The Palms at Palm Springs
572 N. Indian Canyon Dr.
Palm Springs, CA 92262
www.palmsspa.com
Tel: 1-800-753-PALM or 760-325-1111

Post Ranch Inn
Highway 1, P.O. Box 219
Big Sur, CA 93920
Tel: 1-800-527-2200 or 831-667-2200
Fax: 831-667-2824
Website: www.postranchinn.com

Sonoma Mission Inn and Spa
P.O. Box 1447
Sonoma, CA 95476
Tel: 1-800-862-4945 or 707-938-9000
Website: www.sonomamissioninn.com

Two Bunch Palms
67-425 Two Bunch Palms Trail
Desert Hot Springs, CA 92240
Tel: 1-800-472-4334 or 760-323-8791
Fax: 760-323-1317
Website: www.twobunchpalms.com

COLORADO

The Broadmoor
1 Lake Avenue
Colorado Springs, CO 80906
Tel: 1-800-634-7711 or 719-634-7711
Fax: 719-577-5700
Website: www.broadmoor.com

Global Fitness Adventures
P.O. Box 330
Old Snowmass, CO 81654
Tel: 1-800-488-TRIP or 970-927-4793
Fax: 970-927-4793
Website: www.globalfitnessadventures.com

The Lodge and Spa at Cordillera
P.O. Box 1110
Edwards, CO 81632
Tel: 1-800-877-3529 or 970-926-2200
Fax: 970-926-2486
Website: www.cordillera-vail.com

The Peaks Resort & Golden Door Spa
P.O. Box 2702
Telluride Mountain Village, CO 81435
Tel: 1-888-WYN-DHAM or 910-728-6800
Website: www.thepeaksresort.com

Sonnenalp Resort of Vail
20 Vail Road
Vail, CO 81657
Tel: 1-800-654-8312 or 970-476-5656
Fax: 970-476-1639
Website: www.sonnenalp.com

Vail Athletic Club Hotel & Spa
352 E. Meadow Drive
Vail, CO 81657
Tel: 1-800-822-4754 or 970-476-0700
Website: www.vailathleticclub.com

Vail Cascade Club & Spa
1295 Westhaven Drive
Vail, CO 81657
Tel: 1-888-VAIL-SPA or 970-476-7400
Fax: 970-476-7405
Website: www.vailcascade.com

Wyndham Peaks Resort & Golden Door Spa
136 Country Club Drive
Telluride, CO 81435
Tel: 1-800-SPA-KIVA, 1-800-780-2220 or 970-728-6800
Fax: 970-728-6175
Website: www.wyndham.com

CONNECTICUT

The Spa at Norwich Inn
607 West Thames Street
Norwich, CT 06360
Tel: 1-800-ASK4-SPA or 860-886-2401
Website: www.thespaatnorwichinn.com

FLORIDA

Agua at Delano
1685 Collins Avenue
Miami Beach, FL 33139
Tel: 305-673-2900

Eden Roc Resort and Spa
4525 Collins Avenue
Miami Beach, FL 33140
Tel: 305-674-5585
Website: www.edenrocresort.com

Fisher Island Club Spa Internazionale
1 Fisher Island Drive
Fisher Island, FL 33109
Tel: 1-800-537-3708

Professional Golfers Association of America Resort and Spa
400 Avenue of the Champions
Palm Beach Gardens, FL 33418
Tel: 561-624-8400

Regency House Natural Health Spa
2000 South Ocean Drive
Hallandale, FL 33009
Tel: 1-800-454-0003 or 954-454-2220

Sanibel Harbour Resort & Spa
17260 Harbour Pointe Drive
Fort Meyers, FL 33908
Tel: 1-800-767-7777 or 941-466-4000
Fax: 941-466-6050
Website: www.sanibel-resort.com

The Spa at Doral
Doral Golf Resort & Spa
4400 N.W. 87th Avenue
Miami, FL 33178
Tel: 1-800-71-DORAL or 305-591-6471
Fax: 305-591-6480

Spa at the Breakers
One South County Road
Palm Beach, FL 33480
Tel: 1-888 BREAKERS or 561-655-6611
Fax: 561-659-8403

Spa Atlantis Resort & Spa
1460 South Ocean Blvd.
Pompano Beach, FL 33062
Tel: 1-800-583-3500 or 954-941-6688
Fax: 954-943-1219
Website: www.spa-atlantis.com

The Wyndham Resort and Spa
250 Racquet Club Road
Fort Lauderdale, FL 33326
Tel: 954-389-3300
Fax: 954-384-1416
Website: www.wyndham.com

GEORGIA

Sea Island Spa
The Cloister
Sea Island, GA 31561
Tel: 1-800-SEA-ISLAnd

HAWAII

Four Seasons Resort
Hualalai at Historic Ka'upulehu
100 Ka'upulehu-Kona, HI 96740
Tel: 1-800-325-8000
Fax: 1-800-325-8100

Dragonfly Ranch
P.O. Box 675
Honauhau, HW 96726
Tel: 1-800-487-2159 or 808-328-2159
Fax: 808-328-9570
Website: www.dragonflyranch.com

Grand Wailea Resort Hotel & Spa
3850 Wailea Alonui Drive
Waileo, Maui, Hawaii 96753
Tel: 808-875-1234

Hyatt Regency Kauai Resort & Spa
1571 Poipu Road
Kauai, HI 96756
Tel: 808-742-1234
Fax: 808-742-1557

J.W. Marriott Ihilani Resort & Spa at Ko Olina
Ko Olina Resort
92-1001 Olani Street
Kapolei, HW 96707
Tel: 1-808-679-0079
Fax: 808-679-0080
Website: www.ihilani.com

ILLINOIS

Heartland Spa
1237 E. 1600 North Road
Gilman, IL 60938
Tel: 1-800-545-4853
Website: www.heartlandspa.com

INDIANA

Indian Oak Resort & Spa
558 Boundary Road
Chesterton, IN 46304
Tel: 1-800-552-4232 or 219-926-2200
Fax: 219-929-4285
Website: www.indianoak.com

IOWA

The Raj
1754 Jasmine Avenue
Fairfield, IA 52556
Tel: 1-800-248-9050 or 515-472-9580
Fax: 515-472-2496
Website: www.theraj.com

MAINE

Northern Pines Health Retreat
P.O. Box 210
Brownfield, ME 04010
Tel: 207-935-4012
Fax: 207-935-4015
Website: www.maine.com/norpines

MASSACHUSETTS

Canyon Ranch in the Berkshires
165 Kemble Street
Lenox, MA 01240
Tel: 1-800-326-7080 or 413-637-4100
Website: www.canyonranch.com

Kripalu Center for Yoga and Health
P.O. Box 793
West Street, Route 183
Lenox, MA 01240
Tel: 1-800-741-7353 or 413-448-3152
Website: www.kripalu.com

Martha's Vineyard Inn Holistic Retreat & Spa
209 Franklin Street
Vineyard Haven, MA 02568
Tel: 1-800-595-9996 or 508-693-0001
Website: www.mvholisticretreat.com

MICHIGAN

Grand Traverse Resort & Spa
100 Grand Traverse Village Boulevard
Acme, MI 49610
Tel: 1-800-236-1577
Website: www.grandtraverseresort.com

MINNESOTA

Birdwing Spa
21398 575th Avenue
Litchfield, MN 55355
Tel: 320-693-6064
Fax: 320-693-7026

MISSISSIPPI

The Elms Resort & Spa
401 Regent Street
Excelsior Springs, MS 64024
Tel: 1-800-THE-ELMS or 816-630-5500
Fax: 816-630-5380
Website: www.elmsresort.com

NEVADA

Canyon Ranch Spa Club at the Venetian
3355 Las Vegas Boulevard South
Suite 1159
Las Vegas, NV 89109
Tel: 1-877-220-2688 or 702-414-3600

NEW MEXICO

Ten Thousand Waves
P.O. Box 10200
Santa Fe, NM 87504
Tel: 505-992-5025
Fax: 505-989-5077

Vista Clara Ranch Health Spa
H.C. 75, Box 111
Galisteo, NM 87540
Tel: 505-466-4772 or 1-888-NMex-spa
Website: www.vistaclara.com

NEW YORK

Bliss 57
19 E. 57th Street, 3rd floor
New York, NY 10022
Tel: 212-219-8970
Website: www.blissworld.com

Bliss Soho
568 Broadway, 2nd floor
New York, NY 10012
Tel: 212-219-8970
Website: www.blissworld.com

The Copperhood Inn & Spa
Rt. 28
Shandaken, NY 12480
Tel: 845-688-2460
Fax: 845-688-7484
Website: www.copperhood.com

The Emerson Inn & Spa
at Catskill Corners
146 Mount Pleasant Road
Mount Tremper, NY 12457
Tel: 845-688-7900
Fax: 845-688-6789

Gurney's Inn
290 Old Montauk Highway
Montauk, NY
Tel: 1-800-8-GURNEY
Website: www.gurneys-inn.com

Mirror Lake Inn Resort & Spa
5 Mirror Lake Drive
Lake Placid, NY 12946
Tel: 518-523-2544
Fax: 518-523-2871
Website: www.mirrorlakeinn.com

New Age Health Spa
Route 55
Neversink, NY 12765
Tel: 1-800-682-4348 or 845-985-7600
Fax: 845-985-2467
Website: www.newagehealthspa.com

The Sagamore Hotel
on Lake George
Bolton Landing, NY 12814
Tel: 1-800-358-3585 or 518-644-9400

The Stone Spa
104 West 14th Street
New York, NY 10011
Tel: 212-818-1665

NORTH CAROLINA

Westglow European Spa & Resort
2845 Highway 221 South
Blowing Rock, NC 28605
Tel: 1-800-562-0807 or 828-295-4463

OHIO

Kerr House
P.O. Box 363
17777 Beaver Street, Dept. E
Grand Rapids, OH 43522
Tel: 419-832-1733
Fax: 419-832-4303

OREGON

Hickox Salon and Spa
711 S.W. Aldern
Suite 400
Portland, OR 97205
Tel: 503-241-7111

PENNSYLVANIA

Deerfield Spa
650 Resica Falls Road
East Stroudsburg, PA 18301
Tel: 1-800-852-4494 or 570-223-0160
Fax: 570-223-8270

Nemacolin Woodlands Resort & Spa
1001 LaFayette Drive
Farmington, PA 15437
Tel: 1-800-422-2736 or 724-329-8555

SOUTH CAROLINA

Hilton Head Health Institue
14 Valencia Road
Hilton Head Island, SC 29928

Tel: 1-800-292-2440 or 843-785-7292
Fax: 843-686-5659

TENNESSEE

Tennessee Fitness Spa
299 Natural Bridge Park Road
Waynesboro, TN 38485
Tel: 1-800-235-8365
Website: www.TFSpa.com

TEXAS

Four Seasons Resort and Club
Dallas at Las Colinas
4150 North MacArthur Boulevard
Irving, TX 75038
Tel: 972-717-0700
Fax: 972-717-2550
Website: www.fshr.com

The Greenhouse
P.O. Box 1144
Arlington, TX 76004
Tel: 1-800GREENHOUSE or 817-640-4000
Website: www.thegreenhousespa.com

Lake Austin Spa Resort
1705 South Quinlan Park Road
Austin, TX 78732
Tel: 512-372-7300
Fax: 512-266-1572
Website: www.lakeaustin.com

UTAH

Green Valley Resort
1871 West Canyon View Drive
St. George, UT 84770
Tel: 1-800-237-1068 (outside Utah) or
435-628-8060
Fax: 435-673-4084
Website: www.greenvalleyspa.com

Red Mountain Resort & Spa
1275 East Red Mountain Circle
Ivins, UT 84738
Tel: 1-800-407-3002 or 435-673-4905

VERMONT

Green Mountain at Fox Run
P.O. Box 164
Fox Lane

Ludlow, VT 05149
Tel: 1-800-448-8106

New Life Hiking Spa in Killington, VT
The Inn of the Six Mountains
P.O. Box 395
Killington, VT 05751
Tel: 1-800-228-4676
Website: www.newlifehikingspa.com

VIRGINIA

The Homestead
P.O. Box 2000
Hot Springs, VA 24445
Tel: 1-800-838-1766 or 540-839-1766
Website: www.thehomestead.com

WEST VIRGINIA

The Greenbrier in West Virginia
300 West Main Street
White Sulphur Springs, WV 24986
Tel: 1-800-453-4858
Fax: 304-536-7834

WISCONSIN

Grand Geneva Resort and Spa
7036 Grand Geneva Way
Hwy 50 East and 12
Lake Geneva, WI 53147
Tel: 1-800-558-3417 or 262-248-8811
Fax: 262-249-4763
Website: www.grandgeneva.com

WYOMING

Amangani
1535 Northeast Butte Road
Jackson, WY 83001
Tel: 1-877-734-7333 or 307-734-7333
Fax: 307-734-7332

My favorite spas

Spas are as individual as you are–some are great all-rounders while others are best for fitness, pampering, or simply chilling out. With this in mind, we've created this at-a-glance guide to give you a helping hand when you're booking your much deserved spa break. There are, quite literally, hundreds of spas throughout the world (see the spa directory on pages 129 to 136), but this is a selection of some of my personal favorites and those considered to be the best in their particular field. For other spa listings, consult the following:

Spatours
Website: members.aol.com/spatours/spas.htm
SpaAsia
Website: www.spaasia.com
Spa Finder
Website: www.spafinder.com
Tel: 212-924-6800

BEST FOR FITNESS

Australia

The Cape Retreat
Couran Cove Resort Spa and Total Living Centre
Eaglereach Wilderness Resort
Hyatt Regency-Coolum
The Observatory Hotel Spa
The Sanctuary Holistic Retreat
Solar Springs Health Retreat

Canada

Echo Valley Ranch Resort
Mountain Trek Fitness Retreat and Health Spa
Solace Spa at Banff Springs Hotel

The Caribbean

Le Sport

France

Domaine du Royal Club Evian
Institute of Thalassatherapy Louison Bobet

Germany

Brenner's Park Hotel

Indonesia

The Banyan Tree, Bintan

Israel

Carmel Forest Spa Resort

Mexico

Rancho La Puerta

Switzerland

The Grand Hotel and Spa Victoria-Jungfrau

Thailand

The Oriental Spa at The Oriental Bangkok

United Kingdom

The Cowshed at Babington House
Forest Mere Health Farm
Henlow Grange Health Farm
Hoar Cross Hall
Lucknam Park
Ragdale Hall Health Hydro
St David's Hotel and Spa
Stobo Castle Health Spa

United States of America

Agua at Delano
The Ashram
Cal-A-Vie
Canyon Ranch Health Resort
Eden Roc Resort and Spa
Golden Door

Green Valley Fitness Resort and Spa
The Greenhouse
Lake Austin Spa Resort
The Lodge at Skylonda
Ojai Valley Inn and Spa
The Palms at Palm Springs
Professional Golfers Association of America Resort and Spa
The Spa Grande at the Grand Wailea Resort
Vista Clara Ranch Health Spa
Westward Look Resort
The Wyndham Resort and Spa

BEST FOR TRANQUILITY

Australia

Azabu
Daintree Eco-Lodge and Spa
Empire Retreat
The Golden Door Health Retreat
The Observatory Hotel Spa
The Sanctuary Holistic Retreat
Shizuka Ryokan
Solar Springs Health Retreat

Canada

Echo Valley Ranch Resort
Solace Spa at Banff Springs Hotel

The Caribbean

La Casa de Vida Natural
Le Sport

France

Caudalie Institut de Vinotherapie
Domaine du Royal Club Evian
Institute of Thalassatherapy Louison Bobet

Germany

Brenner's Park Hotel

India

The Kairali Ayurvedic Health Resort
The Spa at Rajvilas
The Taj Ayurvedic Centre

Indonesia

The Banyan Tree, Bintan
Jamu Traditional Spa
The Jimbaran Spa at The Four Seasons
Resort
The Mandara Spa at The Chedi
The Mandara Spa at The Ibah
Nusa Dua Beach Hotel and Spa
The Oberoi, Bali
The Oberoi, Lombok
Spa at The Bali Hyatt

Israel

Carmel Forest Spa Resort

Italy

Palazzo Arzaga Spa

Malaysia

The Mandara Spa at The Datai

Mexico

Punta Serena
Rancho La Puerta
The Spa at Las Ventanas al Paradiso

Switzerland

The Grand Hotel and Spa Victoria-
Jungfrau

Thailand

The Banyan Tree, Phuket
Chiva-Som International Health Resort
The Oriental Spa at The Oriental Bangkok

United Kingdom

Champneys at Tring
The Cowshed at Babington House
Forest Mere Health Farm

United States of America

Agua at Delano
The Ashram
Canyon Ranch Health Resort
Eden Roc Resort and Spa
The Expanding Light
Golden Door
Green Valley Fitness Resort and Spa
The Greenhouse
Lake Austin Spa Resort
The Lodge at Skylonda
The Palms at Palm Springs
Ten Thousand Waves
Two Bunch Palms
Vista Clara Ranch Health Spa
Westward Look Resort

BEST FOR ALTERNATIVE TREATMENTS

Australia

Azabu
Daintree Eco-Lodge and Spa
The Sanctuary Holistic Retreat

Canada

Mountain Trek Fitness Retreat and
Health Spa

The Caribbean

La Casa de Vida Natural

India

The Kairali Ayurvedic Health Resort
The Spa at Rajvilas
The Taj Ayurvedic Centre

Indonesia

Jamu Traditional Spa
The Jimbaran Spa at The Four Seasons
Resort
The Mandara Spa at The Chedi
The Oberoi, Bali
The Oberoi, Lombok

Israel

Carmel Forest Spa Resort
Radisson Moriah Plaza Dead Sea Spa Hotel

Mexico

Punta Serena
Rancho La Puerta
The Spa at Las Ventanas al Paradiso

Thailand

The Banyan Tree, Phuket
Chiva-Som International Health Resort

United Kingdom

The Cowshed at Babington House
Forest Mere Health Farm
Ragdale Hall Health Hydro

United States of America

Eden Roc Resort and Spa
The Expanding Light
Golden Door
Ojai Valley Inn and Spa
The Palms at Palm Springs
Vista Clara Ranch Health Spa
Westward Look Resort

BEST FOR PAMPERING

Australia

Azabu
The Cape Retreat
Empire Retreat
The Golden Door Health Retreat
The Sanctuary Holistic Retreat

Canada

Echo Valley Ranch Resort
Solace Spa at Banff Springs Hotel

The Caribbean

La Casa de Vida Natural
Le Sport

France

Caudalie Institut de Vinotherapie
Domaine du Royal Club Evian
Institute of Thalassatherapy Louison Bobet

Germany

Brenner's Park Hotel

India

The Spa at Rajvilas

Indonesia

The Banyan Tree, Bintan
Jamu Traditional Spa
The Jimbaran Spa at The Four Seasons
Resort
The Mandara Spa at The Chedi
The Mandara Spa at The Ibah
Nusa Dua Beach Hotel and Spa
The Oberoi, Bali
The Oberoi, Lombok
Spa at The Bali Hyatt

Israel

Carmel Forest Spa Resort
Radisson Moriah Plaza Dead Sea
Spa Hotel

Italy

Palazzo Arzaga Spa

Mexico

The Spa at Las Ventanas al Paradiso

Switzerland

The Grand Hotel and Spa Victoria-
Jungfrau

Thailand

The Banyan Tree, Phuket
Chiva-Som International Health Resort
The Oriental Spa at The Oriental
Bangkok

United Kingdom

Agua at Sanderson
Henlow Grange Health Farm
Hoar Cross Hall
Ragdale Hall Health Hydro
St David's Hotel and Spa
Stobo Castle Health Spa

United States of America

The Ashram
Canyon Ranch Health Resort
Eden Roc Resort and Spa
The Expanding Light
Green Valley Fitness Resort and Spa
Lake Austin Spa Resort
The Lodge at Skylonda
Ojai Valley Inn and Spa
The Palms at Palm Springs
Professional Golfers Association of
America Resort and Spa
The Spa Grande at the Grand Wailea
Resort
Ten Thousand Waves
Two Bunch Palms
Westward Look Resort
The Wyndham Resort and Spa

BEST FOR FOOD

Australia

Daintree Eco-Lodge and Spa
The Golden Door Health Retreat
Hyatt Regency-Coolum
The Observatory Hotel Spa

Canada

Solace Spa at Banff Springs Hotel

France

Domaine du Royal Club Evian

India

The Spa at Rajvilas

Indonesia

The Banyan Tree, Bintan
Nusa Dua Beach Hotel and Spa
The Oberoi, Bali
The Oberoi, Lombok

Italy

Palazzo Arzaga Spa

Malaysia

The Mandara Spa at The Datai

Mexico

Rancho La Puerta
The Spa at Las Ventanas al Paradiso

Switzerland

The Grand Hotel and Spa Victoria-
Jungfrau

Thailand

The Oriental Spa at The Oriental
Bangkok

United Kingdom

Agua at Sanderson
Henlow Grange Health Farm
Hoar Cross Hall
Lucknam Park
St David's Hotel and Spa
Stobo Castle Health Spa

United States of America

The Ashram
Canyon Ranch Health Resort
Eden Roc Resort and Spa
The Expanding Light
Green Valley Fitness Resort and Spa
Lake Austin Spa Resort
The Lodge at Skylonda
The Spa Grande at the Grand Wailea
Resort
Ten Thousand Waves
Two Bunch Palms
Westward Look Resort

Home-spa suppliers

Aveda
Tel: 612-783-4000 for suppliers
Beauty products inspired by ancient ayurvedic know-how, including body cleansers, skin creams, toners, and scented candles.

Bach Flower Remedies
Tel: 978-988-3833 for suppliers
Flower remedies including the acclaimed Rescue Remedy, useful for treating emotional problems and stress.

Bath and Body Works
Tel: 614-856-6000 for suppliers
Fantastic selection of body scrubs, scented candles, bath treats, and accessories at budget prices.

Borghese
Tel: 212-659-5300 for suppliers
Famous for therapeutic spa-style mineral muds, body scrubs, and mineral-enriched face and body preparations originating from the renowned Montecatini region of Italy.

Caudalie
Tel: 212-695-4400 for suppliers
Grape-based skin preparations for bath, body, and face from the French "Grape Vine" Spa.

Crabtree & Evelyn
Tel: 860-928-2761 for suppliers
Purveyors of spa-style face and body products, scented candles, and aromatherapy-based preparations.

Coty
Tel: 212-479-4300 for suppliers
The "Healing Garden" range includes bath products, incense sticks, scented candles, and sprays–all of which contain botanical extracts.

Elemis
Tel: 1-800-496-0201 for suppliers
Premium quality, plant-based face and body preparations used at over 300 spas internationally.

E'Spa
Tel: 212-250-0100 for suppliers
Used in some of the world's most exclusive spas, the E'Spa range includes soothing skin treatments, seaweed-enriched bath preparations, and aromatherapy-based bath and body oils.

Kiehl's, Inc.
Tel: 1-800-543-4571 for suppliers
Fragrance oils, unscented shampoos, beauty and body products.

L'Occitane
Tel: 888-623-2880 for suppliers
For delicious aromatherapy oils, foam baths, bath salts, candles, body brushes, and soaps.

Origins
Tel: 212-219-9764 for suppliers
Face and body products with naturally derived skin-enhancing ingredients, including the legendary Salt Rub body scrub, Liquid Clay foaming cleanser, and Soothing Sea Salts for the bath. Wide selection of body brushes and bath mitts.

Sephora
Tel: 212-944-6789 for suppliers
Emporium of fragrances, cosmetics, and skincare products, offering a wide selection from hard-to-find brands and classic names to their own Sephora Collection.

The Body Shop
Tel: 919-554-4900
International retailer of skin and hair products, aromatherapy treatments, and bath and body products.

Tisserand
Tel: 707-769-5120 for suppliers
Excellent quality essential oils and aromatherapy-based products.

Zenith Supplies, Inc.
Tel: 1-800-735-7217 for suppliers
Essential oils, botanical products

DIRECT FROM THE SPA . . .

Experience a taste of the spa lifestyle with the following home-spa products.

Mandara Spa
Tel: +62 361 755 575 or e-mail jmatthews@mandaraspa.com
Beautiful range of Mandara Massage Oils, soaps, bath, and body products.

Nusa Dua Beach Hotel and Spa
Tel: +62 361 771210 or
e-mail ndbhnet@indosat.net.id.
The Esens range of spa products created by spa consultants Kim and Cary Collier includes a DIY Lalur Kit, one-shot massage oils, and luxurious bath preparations. Also available direct from Esens, tel: +62 361 771 991 or e-mail Collierspas@hotmail.com.

Westward Look Resort
Tel: 520-297-0134 or check out www.westwardlook.com for further details
Try the Revitalizer Kit, which includes a Westward Look robe and Sensi massage sandals, and the Stress Relief Bath Therapy Kit, which includes massage and body oil, bath salts, and natural sea sponge. A wide selection of herbal and bath teas are also available.

Further reading

BATHROOMS

Bathroom by Suzanne Ardley (Dorling Kindersley)
Essence of White by Hilary Mandleberg (Hearst Books)
Pure Style by Jane Cumberbatch (Stewart, Tabori & Chang)
The Sensual Home by Ilse Crawford (Rizzoli)

RELAXATION

The Bloomsbury Encyclopaedia of Aromatherapy by Chrissie Wildwood (Inner Traditions)
The Complete illustrated Guide to Yoga by Howard Kent (Element)
Tree of Yoga by B.K.S. Iyengar (Shambhala Pubns)

SPA FOOD

Canyon Ranch Cooking – Bringing the Spa Home by Jeanne Jones (Harper Collins)
The Golden Door Cookbook by Michel Stroot (Broadway)
Great Tastes – Healthy Cooking From Canyon Ranch (Canyon Ranch)
The Rancho La Puerta Cookbook by Bill Wavrin (Broadway)

FACE AND BODY TREATS

The Book of Ayurveda by Judith H. Morrison (Fireside)
Indian Beauty Secrets by Monisha Bharadwaj (Ulysses Press)
The Tropical Spa by Sophie Benge (Periplus)

Index

Acknowledgments

A massive thank-you to the following for their contributions to this project.

Researcher Kate Hames for all her hard work, faxing, e-mailing and phone calling around the globe.

My best-mate-down-under, Melinda Aldridge for all her assistance and persistence on the Aussie front.

And the following photographers: Brian Nice, for his beautiful and inspiring images, endless Fed Ex packages and transatlantic support; Simon Brown, for allowing us to use his gorgeous bathroom and bathing pictures; Stefano Massimo for permitting us to use some of his wonderful photographs.

Denise Bates, for her constant support, endless patience, and serenity–even when the going was tough!

Emma Callery, for her attention to detail, wonderful editing, and overall loveliness throughout.

Ciara Lunn, for keeping up with it all and tracking me down when needed!

Helen Lewis, for her inspirational design.

Carol Pullen, for the inspiration, endless cups of Rosie Lee, and for keeping me motivated when my energy was flagging.

Sue, Hazel, and Frances Sherar, for all the moral support and encouragement, not to mention the long walks!

Thanks to all at New Romney Junior and Infants Schools for their constant support, especially Michele Rowland, Mrs Brown, Mrs Haldane, and all their pupils.

Huge thanks also goes to the following people for their help, contributions, recipes, and shared secrets: Belinda Shepherd at The Four Seasons; Sue Arnett in the public relations department for Rancho La Puerta and Golden Door; Katie Garber at Canyon Ranch; Mary Beth Chambers at Lake Austin Spa Resort; Marilyn Carr at The Expanding Light; Donna Kreutz at the Westward Look Resort; Merrill Williams at Ojai Valley Inn and Spa; Annie Kinnane at the Couran Cove Resort; Norman Dove at Echo Valley Ranch Resort, Canada; Clare and Caroline at Ann Scott Associates, London; Clare Branch at St David's Hotel & Spa; Anne Hart at Henlow Grange; Gillie Turner at Champneys; Angela Hopkins at the Hyatt Regency Coolum; Belinda Anderson at The Golden Door Health Retreat, Australia; Veda Dante at Daintree Eco Lodge & Spa; Vicki Taylor at Ragdale Hall; fitness expert Dean Hodgkin; Mr Yasin Zargar at Indus Tours and Travel Ltd; John Wallwork and Michael Jacques at T'ai Chi UK, tel: +44 (0)20 7407 4775 or visit the website at www.taichiuk.co.uk; Sean Harrington from Elemis; Sue Harmsworth from E'Spa; Leila Fazel at Agua; Lydia Sarfati at Repechage.

The copyright for the Native Body Glow recipe on page 86 rests with Vista Clara Ranch Health Spa.

The publishers thank the following photographers and organizations for the photographs that appear in this book

Page 1 Stefano Massimo, 2 Brian Nice, 4 top Brian Nice, 4 bottom Craig Robertson, 7 Brian Nice, 8 Arcaid (Richard Powers), 10 Simon Brown, 13 Simon Brown, 17 x 4 Simon Brown, 20 Simon Brown, 24 Brian Nice, 29 Brian Nice, 33 Tony Stone Images (Andrea Booher), 36 x 4 Retna (Philip Reeson), 44 Craig Robertson, 49 Craig Robertson, 56 Craig Robertson, 61 Craig Robertson, 64 Craig Robertson, 68 Stefano Massimo, 71 Brian Nice, 72 Brian Nice, 75 top left Tony Stone Images (Laurent Monneret), 75 top right, bottom left and right Brian Nice, 76 Brian Nice, 84 Brian Nice, 89 x 4 Simon Brown, 93 Brian Nice, 97 Brian Nice, 98 Brian Nice, 101 x 4 Simon Brown, 104 Brian Nice, 109 Brian Nice, 111 Brian Nice, 112 top left and right, bottom right Simon Brown, 112 bottom left PWA, 116 Brian Nice, 121 Brian Nice, 125 Stefano Massimo, 128 Stefano Massimo.

All illustrations by Lynne Robinson